Tommy V Cancer
One Man's Battle Against The Big C
Tommy Donbavand

Published worldwide by Serpo Books

www.tommydonbavand.com
www.tommyvcancer.com
www.patreon.com/tommydonbavand

Cover artwork © 2017 by Nigel Parkinson
www.nigelparkinsoncartoons.blogspot.co.uk

To Kirsty, Arran and Sam
&
Bryan and Sue
for always being by my side

COMING UP...

I t was dark.

And not just 'absence of light' dark. It was as though someone had thrown the darkness over me, smothering me in the inability to see. Or even think.

I was aware that there were people nearby. I couldn't tell what they were saying (their voices seemed to be coming from many miles away), but I could tell that they were agitated.

They sounded worried about something.

Then, one of the voices broke through...

"Thomas. Thomas, can you hear me?"

"Yes," I replied.

"Can you open your eyes, Thomas?"

I tried, but couldn't, and told the disembodied voice as much.

"OK," he said. "Do you know where you are right now?"

This one gave me pause to think for a moment. "No," I admitted. "I don't know where I am."

"Thomas, you're in A&E."

I think I actually chuckled then. "No, I'm not!" I said. "Why would I be in A&E?"

And that was it. The voice faded away to mix with the general hubbub and chatter of background noise. The conversation was, apparently, over.

I didn't find out until later, but this conversation was taking place in the resuscitation room at Blackburn Hospital while doctors fought to save my life

I had, apparently, fallen out of bed in the early hours of the morning and Kirsty had been unable to wake me up. First one, then two ambulance crews were called to carry me downstairs to the gleaming yellow chariot that was to speed me to A&E and then the Intensive Care Unit.

At that point, the doctors took my family aside and told them that, unless I started responding very soon, I had approximately two hours left to live.

ABOUT THIS BOOK

This book began life as a blog. A blog I kept to chart the course of my journey through diagnosis, treatment and recuperation.

As such, each 'chapter' is a separate blog entry and therefore some are much shorter than others.

I've removed the date stamps from most of the entries, but kept them for important events, such as the treatment sessions and hospital stays.

Please bear in mind that a lot of these blog entries were written when I was in pain, depressed, scared - or all three at once. As a result, there are places where you are unlikely to experience my best writing.

It's tough to keep on top of your craft when you're terrified that the next day could well be your last.

ABOUT THE AUTHOR

Tommy Donbavand is the author of over 100 books for young readers, including the 13-title *Scream Street* series, which has now been adapted as a stop-motion animated TV show for CBBC and other channels worldwide.

He has also written *Doctor Who: Shroud of Sorrow*, *My Teacher Ate My Brain*, *Dinner Ladies of Dooooooom!* and many more books especially for reluctant and struggling readers. His other books include series such as *Fangs: Vampire Spy*, *Snow-Man*, *Time Trek*, and *Space Hoppers*.

In comics and magazines, Tommy writes the regular comic strip in the monthly science mag for kids, *Whizz, Pop, Bang!*, fun National Curriculum based content for *Amazing!*, and he is proud to write for his favourite ever weekly comic, *The Beano*, where he provides the adventures for classic characters such as *Bananaman* and *The Bash Street Kids*. He has also written scripts and stories for the Twelfth Doctor and The Paternoster Gang in *Doctor Who Adventures*.

When not writing, Tommy can be found thinking about writing, looking forward to writing, and feeling relieved that he has finished writing for the day. On the rare occasion where writing is not occupying his mind, he enjoys playing guitar and harmonica, and making balloon animals - although not all at the same time.

Tommy lives in Lancashire, England with his wife, two sons and a seemingly endless stream of pets.

INTRODUCTION

On Thursday, 10th of March 2016, I returned home from a hospital appointment and broke the news to my wife and children. I had throat cancer. Stage four. Inoperable.

Desperately needing some way to make sense of my situation, I set up a blog to chart my battle against the disease. I hoped it would allow me to understand more about this thing inside me, and what I would have to go through in terms of treatment to try to eradicate it. I also thought it might help other people who found themselves in similar circumstances.

I made a promise to my readers to be open and honest all the way. I wouldn't hold anything back, no matter how unpleasant.

Now, over a year later, I have adapted that blog into this book. It details my journey from when I first realised that something was wrong, through the intense courses of chemotherapy and radiotherapy, to where I am today. To say that journey was difficult is a vast understatement.

The side effects of my treatment utterly kicked my arse,

causing me to lose over half my bodyweight and fall seriously ill with double pneumonia and sepsis. Totally unresponsive, I was rushed into intensive care where the doctors told my family that, if they couldn't stabilise me, I had approximately two hours left to live. One option was to put me into a medically induced coma, although the chances were high that I would never emerge from it.

Imagine someone telling you that about your loved one as they lie there, unconscious and struggling to breathe. Cancer is an invader that affects more than just the patient. Everyone suffers - spouses, siblings, children, extended family, friends. Even, as I was to discover, strangers from all over the world. I was overwhelmed with the love and kindness of almost everyone who contacted me, but I also suffered terrible abuse at the hands of online trolls.

I should warn you that parts of this book do not make for easy reading. I kept my promise to be honest, and wrote many of the blog entries when I was depressed and scared, certain I wouldn't live to see another dawn. I convinced myself that I would quickly perish, leaving my wife and two sons - then aged 9 and 17 - alone, and with no-one to protect them or provide for them.

I wouldn't get to see them grow up, develop into young men, and eventually have children of their own. The prospect terrified me.

For those of you who followed my blog and read the posts as I uploaded them, you haven't seen everything. This book contains plenty of new content, including updates from when I was either in hospital or simply too ill to write. I also explain how I'm coping now, and the ways in which my life has changed forever.

Cancer is pure, unadulterated evil. I lost both of my parents to the disease (my dad less than a year before my story begins). And now the bastard had come for me. I was in for one hell of a fight.

Tommy Donbavand, July 2017

MUMPS

My doctor thought I had mumps.

This was back in November 2015. I'd been suffering with a sore throat and what I suspected was a swollen gland for a couple of weeks, and it wasn't getting any better.

I had a week-long book tour of Guernsey fast approaching, so I wanted to get on top of things before I set off. I didn't fancy tackling two or three schools a day - plus several evening events - with a bad throat.

At this point, I should admit that I hadn't been in the best of health for a few years. I was very overweight, and had chronic asthma - the combination of which usually resulted in either a throat or a chest infection at least twice a year. March and October were the months to bet on if you liked a flutter.

However, in recent years, my body had decided that a mere chest infection wasn't good enough. No, it had traded the chest infections in and upgraded to pneumonia. And, on special occasions, pneumonia and pleurisy combined.

I'd been hospitalised four times over the past three years with those buggers!

But, that hadn't been a problem for a while. My last stint in hospital (once more with the winning team of pneumonia and pleurisy) had been in March 2015. Since then, I'd been reasonably good at breathing and not needing an ambulance.

Then I got this sore throat, and the swelling. So, I went to see my doctor (and - for the first time in six years - actually saw my own doctor!)

"It's mumps!" she said, gently prodding at the lump in my neck. "I could tell the second you walked in through the door."

"Can you give me anything for that?"

"No, it will go down by itself. But, I have to warn you that this will take a while."

She wasn't wrong about the last part...

SCHOOL VISITS

As part of my job, I've always visited a lot of schools each year to teach creative writing and instil a love of reading for pleasure. These visits provided a healthy portion of my income. Not all authors are paid on the JK Rowling sliding scale; most of us just about make enough to live on.

And not just schools – there are also libraries and book festivals, too. One of my favourites is the *Edinburgh International Book Festival*, which I've performed at on several occasions.

School visits are great fun, but the thing about them is that schools are full of kids.

Smelly, snotty, grimy, noisy kids.

I love 'em! The feedback you can get on your ideas in a primary school classroom is better than anything you'll ever receive from an editor.

But, they're full of germs! Kids, that is, not editors.

Well, not all of them.

And that's where I caught coughs and colds every now and then. In schools. From kids.

Mind you, teachers don't help... "line up, then you can all shake Tommy's hand on the way out!"

Shudder!

Coughs, colds, flu, throat infections, chest infections. I've caught them all.

In fact, back in 2009, I picked up swine flu at a school visit!

So that's why being diagnosed with mumps didn't seem strange to me. I'd obviously picked up the bugger during a school visit.

And, we were coming up to World Book Day - the one day in March each year when head teachers remember that authors exist and ALL try to book you in for a visit in the same week. I had a LOT of school visits lined up in the early part of 2016, including the aforementioned trip to Guernsey, where I was due to visit 15 different schools over just 5 days.

I hoped to get better before that madness started. But, I didn't.

I got worse.

The pain increased, and the lump grew in size.

And I started to lose weight.

Oh, shit.

BLOOD TEST

OK, something wasn't right. So, I went back to see the doctor.

I was told I had a throat infection, and possibly an infected lymph node.

Another week went by, and I was still in a lot of pain. The lump was still increasing in size, and I was getting rather concerned.

This time, the doctor did a thorough examination, then went to talk to a senior doctor, who also did a thorough examination. And then they took some blood.

I say some blood; they took pints of the stuff! And that's not easy to do with me as I have very small, almost invisible veins. The two doctors had to summon a nurse to try and take the blood after they had each failed more than once to find a vein.

Eventually, they got the blood they needed without wringing me dry. And a letter was sent to the Ear, Nose and Throat Department at Blackburn Hospital, asking for an appointment with a consultant.

Now it wasn't just me who was concerned...

FAMILY GUY

I'm very lucky to have a close family around me - in both my wife and children, and my extended family. Which is why I wanted to tell them that there might be a problem sooner, rather than later.

You see, both of my parents died from cancer.

My mum - Elizabeth Mary Donbavand - died from lung cancer in December 2005.

My dad - Brian Thomas Donbavand - died from prostate cancer which had spread to his bones in June, 2015.

I was able to discuss my worries and fears with my wife Kirsty, of course. My brother and sister were obviously concerned when they heard the news, and they asked that I keep them updated. Plus, the lump was really showing by now. They couldn't have missed it.

Then it came to my children - Sam (9) and Arran (16).

What on earth do you say to kids in these situations? I wanted to be honest with them; they'd both be hurt if I lied to them, even if it was to protect their feelings.

Plus, Sam suffers from Asperger's Syndrome, and he processes information in a different way to the rest of us. He can get upset at the slightest hint of change in his life - and this might be a biggie. I'd have to be cunning...

So, I told them I had *Schrodinger's Lump*.

You might know the story of *Schrodinger's Cat* - a scientist placed a cat inside a lead box, along with a vial of poison. While the box remained locked, there was no way to tell whether the cat had broken open the vial and, therefore, whether the cat was dead or alive. As a result, scientists decided that the cat was both dead and alive at the same time.

I sat the boys down, and explained about the lump, and how much pain it was causing me. I gave it the name *Schrodinger's Lump* because it might be something serious, but it also might not be something serious.

Therefore, we agreed that the lump was both a concern, but nothing to panic about until I had undergone further tests.

I don't know who that conversation helped more - me, or my kids.

DIAGNOSIS WAS MURDER

"It's not good news..."

Those were the words spoken by the consultant at the ENT clinic in Blackburn Hospital. That was the moment I knew I had cancer.

Actually, I'd known a few minutes earlier when my wife and I were called in to get the results of my biopsy. Instead of just the consultant and the nurse in the room, as before, now there was a third person. A woman with a very serious expression on her face. And she was clutching a clipboard.

Nothing good ever comes on clipboards.

That was when I knew.

Although, to be fair, I'd suspected what the diagnosis would be when the receptionist in the X-ray department booked in for a CT scan for the next day. Appointments usually take weeks, at the very least. Hurrying a scan wasn't a good sign.

Neither was the fact that the consultant had taken FOUR samples during my biopsy – two from the outside of the lump in my throat/neck, and two from inside. The complete right hand side of my face and neck had been numbed, and then the consultant had slid open a drawer of tools that wouldn't look out of place of the set of a horror movie. They glinted in the harsh, fluorescent light. If they had voices, they would have been cackling.

The first two samples were taken via a gadget that was pressed against my throat, then a thin saw punctured my skin and slid inside my lump. It was horrible – not because I could feel the samples being taken, but because I could hear the saw rasping back and forth on the flesh inside, well... inside me!

I can't even be in the kitchen when my wife cuts up pieces of chicken!

The two inner samples were simply ripped out of the lump. By that point, I had a weird feeling that something was amiss. This feeling was enhanced by the consultant's insistence that I didn't go home but, instead, returned for the biopsy results in 45 minutes' time.

That was a fun three-quarters of an hour, I can tell you.

But, does it really matter? Does it matter if I can pin down the exact moment when I knew I had cancer? Is that in the slightest bit important?

I really don't know. After three failed attempts, the radiographer finally managed to find a vein, and the dye was injected in. Then, I had to lie back while the CT scanner whirred into life above my head.

I almost cried then.

Not because I was scared of the scan, but because I suddenly realised that this was going to be my life for the foreseeable future. Whatever the results of this scan are (I find out on Tuesday), it will mean some form of treatment is put in place. Treatment that will require frequent hospital trips, tests, scans and who knows what else.

My world has changed.

SCAN THE MAN

As I write this, it's 9pm on Monday 14th March 2016. In 17 hours' time - at 2pm tomorrow - I will get the results of my CT scan. I'll find out how far the cancer has spread through my body, and what my treatment will be.

Friends have emailed to ask how I'm feeling.

The best reply would be - numb.

I've felt that way since the consultant told me that I had cancer. It was as though all the colour was suddenly washed out of the world.

I realised that I could hear someone crying, and was very surprised to discover that it wasn't me.

It was Kirsty.

I was suddenly overwhelmed with the dreadful feeling that I had let her and the boys down.

"Will it happen soon?" I asked the lady with the clipboard.

"Will what happen soon?"

"He's asking if he's going to die soon," Kirsty explained.

"We don't know," admitted the lady.

I wish I could remember her name, she was very kind.

Back in the waiting room I sent text messages to my brother and sister to tell them the result of the biopsy, and asked them not to call yet as I would have to gather myself together enough so that I could drive home (Kirsty doesn't drive. She might have to learn).

As I walked across the car park with Kirsty, hand in hand, I discovered another feeling. I felt relieved that my Mum and Dad weren't here to hear the bad news. It would upset them so much.

NEWS JUST IN

I've just arrived home from the hospital, where I got the results from Friday's CT scan. That was an anxious wait, let me tell you!

Apparently, the cancer started in my tonsils and the base of my tongue, and has now spread to the right hand side of my throat. Nowhere else is affected as yet.

The lump is too big for surgery, so I start six week courses (approx.) of both chemotherapy and radiotherapy next week. I had to have my teeth x-rayed today as any potential dental problems can be worsened by the effects of the chemo and/or radiotherapy.

Who knew?

Now, here comes the fun part...

I'm going to need a feeding tube put directly into my stomach to be able to eat as swallowing will be too painful...

...and a dedicated course of speech therapy afterwards as I'm likely to have trouble talking once my throat has been nuked for six weeks straight.

Yikes!

Those last two points aside, it's not as bad as I'd feared.

I'll be honest and admit that I was certain the consultant would tell me that the cancer had reached my brain. But it hasn't.

Yet.

And that's a good thing.

I suppose I'd better start thinking about a style of hat to wear for when my hair goes. That's actually trickier than it sounds as there are a lot of hats out there that instantly make me look like a serial killer as soon as I put them on. I can't do anything woollen, and the peaked baseball cap just isn't a good match.

PLAIN PAIN

I t hurts tonight. Right across the side of my throat and neck where the lump is, and up the side of my face past my right ear.

I've taken my painkillers - but they don't seem to be kicking in. At least, not yet. I was surviving on soluble paracetamol and codeine, but then the doctor gave me something called Tramadol. It's supposed to be stronger, but I can't say I've really noticed.

I tried to go to bed an hour ago in the hope that I could sleep it off. No such luck. I just couldn't get comfortable, no matter how I tossed and turned. So, I'm up again.

When it feels like this, I'm reminded just how bad my situation is.

Don't get me wrong, I know it could be a lot worse. The doctors say they have caught the cancer reasonably early, and before it has spread too far.

But that doesn't change the fact that, as I sit here, I have one of the deadliest diseases known to man inside my head!

Just think about that for a second.

I carry this thing around with me, 24 hours a day, 7 days a

week - inside my skull. I provide it with a warm, moist environment in which to survive, grow and feed.

I'm feeding this bastard! This monster inside my own head.

Does it have a plan? I assume that, if it were to be left unchecked, that it would continue to spread - but does it decide where to go next, or does it just take the path of least resistance?

I'm terrified it will reach my brain.

And that's not such a leap, considering it already shares the same container as my grey matter.

I wish I could reach inside and just rip it out.

I suppose that's what surgery is, in the end. A controlled way of ripping the beast out from inside me. But my growth is already too big to be operated on. I wonder if it knows that.

I wonder if it feels safe.

But, of course, it's not safe. At some point within the next ten days, it will be under attack from both radiotherapy and chemotherapy. Or, to be more exact, we both will. Attacking just the cancer alone would be like trying to fry an egg while leaving the shell intact.

I'm a shell.

I protect this f*cking thing from harm.

The radio waves will have to pass through me to get to this thing. The chemicals will have to scour the inside of my body, searching for it.

It's going to hurt, and I'm scared.

Really scared.

I've tried to stay calm and not admit that to anyone, but it's true. I'm just as terrified of the treatment as I am of the disease it will try to eradicate.

Will the cancer be scared, too?

Once it is under attack, will any kind of self-preservation

kick in? Even on the most basic level, all living organisms want to stay that way - alive. Is it any different for living organisms we don't like?

This sounds mad, and maybe it's the effect of the painkillers talking here, but they say babies in the womb can pick up on the feelings and emotions of their mothers. Will this be the same?

Is this thing my baby?

Time and time again, people have told me to stay positive, and not to give in. Positive thinking is the key. I will beat the cancer. I must beat the cancer.

If it had independent thought, would the cancer be thinking the same thing about the treatment I'm about to undergo?

I wonder what colour it is. I really don't want to know, but ridiculous questions like that keep popping into my head.

You know - the head I now share with another living entity.

I know I could Google it and see plenty of pictures of various forms of cancer, but I can't imagine anything worse, to be honest. That would terrify me to a degree I don't even want to think about.

I tried to joke about it today. I told my wife that it wasn't cancer, but a second brain developing. An internal back-up drive where I could dump random knowledge, leaving space in my main brain for new story ideas.

We laughed at that. Together.

We laughed at the cancer inside my head.

Damn, this thing hurts!

LOVE THE NHS

I've just returned home from an appointment with my GP - Dr Ellison. She's fantastic. So kind and caring - and she's into many of the same things as me, including *Doctor Who* and *The Beano*! I should point out here that she's *not* the doctor who mis-diagnosed my cancer as mumps!

A few years ago, I made her a character in my *Doctor Who* novel, *Shroud of Sorrow* (she's Dr Ellison at Parkland Memorial Hospital in Dallas). And, more recently, she made a cameo appearance in *The Bash Street Kids*.

Today, however, she led me through the results of my CT scan, answered my questions, swapped my pain relief from Tramadol to morphine, and prescribed some sleeping tablets.

And she gave me a big hug as I was leaving.

Told you - fantastic!

In fact, everyone I've seen over the course of this diagnosis has been amazing. Thank whichever deity you believe in for the NHS (for non-UK readers, the National Health Service), and the amazing people who work there.

On the day of my biopsy, junior doctors were on strike

here in the UK (if you don't know why, you should look it up - they're being shafted by rhyming-slang named health minister and a Tory government out to fill their own pockets).

I beeped the car horn as I drove past the picket line, and gave them all a thumbs up. They work so hard to keep people like me in good health, and then treat us when things go wrong.

The way they are being dealt with is very unfair, as is this government's slow and sly privatisation of the NHS. But, that's a blog post for another day...

I'm about to undergo some serious treatment and, thanks to that rarest of all creatures - a politician with a soul - I won't be faced with a huge bill afterwards.

Which is just as well, as I'd be rubbish at making Crystal Meth!

That politician was the Labour Minister of Health from 1945 to 1951 - Nye Bevan. The man who founded the NHS.

And we should all be thankful.

Ten years ago, my Mum spent a week in a coma in the Intensive Care Unit at Chorley Hospital before she died. One day, when we arrived to visit her, we discovered that one of the nurses had washed her hair and tied it back with a white ribbon.

She didn't have to do that. That's not part of her job description. My Mum didn't even know about it. But it made all the difference to a family who were about to lose one of their loved ones.

A few months later, the unit held a chapel service to remember everyone who had passed away over the last year. We signed a book of thanks afterwards, and I'll always remember what my Dad wrote in it...

'I'm not religious, and I don't believe in God but, a few

months ago, I met angels. They were disguised as doctors and nurses.'

So please, please remember that we have to support the NHS and its incredible staff at every opportunity.

I'll climb down from my soapbox now!

I have a few pieces of writing to work on today: a new script for *The Bash Street Kids*, two short books in my new reluctant reader series for *Badger Learning*, and a chapter of the first book in my new children's horror series for *Oxford University Press*.

Tomorrow, I'm hoping to pop in to the school I was due to visit on World Book Day, but had to cancel as I was just too unwell. I doubt I'll be able to run any creative writing workshops or give my usual author talk, but it will be great to see all the pupils. From what I hear, they've been making *Scream Street* masks to show me!

Life, it appears, goes on...

SEE THE LITTLE PIXIES

Wahey!

Morphine's great, isn't it?

Me and all the little dancing pixies think so, anyway.

I'm joking, of course.

The pixies stopped dancing once the flying badgers turned up.

At least my face and throat doesn't hurt as much, which is a good thing. As are all the wonderful messages I've been getting from people around the world. Some from friends, others from strangers. All very welcome.

I've come to realise that people who talk to you about your cancer fall into one of two groups...

- A - the people who want to wish you well.
- B - the people who want to wish you well by telling you, in graphic detail, about the time their brother/niece/cousin/boss/neighbour had cancer - and the horrendous time they had to endure through treatment and/or surgery.

Still, they mean well.

I need a haircut.

Ha!

A haircut! Is it worth the trouble if I'm likely to lose it anyway? That reminds me... I still haven't settled on a style of hat in case that happens.

Now, where was I?

Oh, yeah...

Morphine's great, isn't it?

SCHOOL'S OUT

Today I visited Broadoak Primary School in Ashton-Under-Lyne. I was originally supposed to be there on World Book Day (3rd March), but I couldn't go as I was in the early stages of my tests.

Then I rearranged the visit for Wednesday (two days ago), but my throat was so closed up that I could barely talk. So, I went today.

It was hard. Very hard.

When I visit a school, I usually run a series of creative writing workshops for the pupils, then get everyone together in the hall to give my hour-long author talk, describing how I became an author in a fun, interactive way.

Yesterday, I couldn't do those things.

I ran four sessions with different year groups, talking about my career with the help of a PowerPoint presentation - and that pushed my ability to talk aloud to the very limit. My throat kept catching, and I had a lot of difficulty pronouncing certain words and phrases - including, rather unhelpfully, 'Scream Street'.

By the time I left the school at 3.30pm, my throat was ragged. I was in a lot of pain.

I won't be able to do any more schools until I'm 100% over this. Which is a big problem.

Visiting schools makes up half of my income, and cancer has taken that away in one go. That's a terrifying thought.

Plus, finances aside, I love school visits. I love helping pupils with their creative writing and making them laugh from the moment I arrive. I love inspiring reluctant readers to give one of my books a try, and then receiving emails from them afterwards saying how much they've enjoyed reading for the very first time. Visiting schools is an incredible thing to do with your time.

In the past ten years, I've visited at least 70 schools a year.

700 school visits.

And cancer has taken all that away from me, too. For the foreseeable future, at least.

As if I didn't hate it enough already.

But, it wasn't all bad. I came away from Broadoak piled high with thank you and get well cards - and an amazing *Scream Street* hat, courtesy of the pupils in year 5.

It could be the one to wear when my hair goes.

GET DOWN

I t's 3.15pm, and I've just got out of bed.

I tried to get up earlier - several times - but I just couldn't do it.

I couldn't face it.

The enormity of what I'm about to go through hit me in the night and I just sank into a black hole of worry.

How will I cope with the impending treatment? What will happen if the treatment isn't successful? Will this leave me susceptible to another attack in years to come?

Most of you won't know that - in addition to my asthma and now the cancer, I also suffer from clinical depression. I've been on anti-depressants for years now, and they're working well.

Or, at least, they were.

When I saw my doctor the other day, she assured me that this wasn't a death sentence. But, she did discuss the danger of the cancer spreading further from its current location. If it goes lower, it could attack my larynx - and that could result in surgery that would render me mute.

If it goes higher, it approaches my brain.

She said I'm lucky it has developed exactly where it is.

I don't feel lucky.

I spent most of the night running worst case scenarios through my mind. How Kirsty and the boys would cope without me. Worrying that they would have to move house.

That could mean Sam moving to a new school and Arran to a different college. I'd hate that to happen. They're so happy where they are now.

I told Kirsty that I want her to meet someone else. Someone who can look after them all. Better than I can right now.

Shit. Crying now. Sorry.

I know this is my depression kicking in, and that I can't let it. If I start spiralling down, I'll lose the fight inside me. I'll lose my anger at this thing and my resolve to beat it.

My mum used to call it my bounce. When I was low, she used to tell me to get my bounce back.

I wish I could talk to her now. My Dad, too. I'm terrified of going through this without them. But, I'll have to.

I was an adult when I lost my parents to cancer and it tore me apart, both times. How will the boys cope if they lose me? They're just kids.

I'm not a religious man. I used to be, but not anymore.

I was brought up a Catholic. In my teens, I was really into it. I played guitar at folk mass each week, and was part of a religious group at school. As I grew up, my beliefs began to melt away - but there was always something there. In the background.

Until my mum died.

I lost it all that day. As if someone had flipped a switch.

Click. Gone. Forever.

Don't get me wrong. I don't preach atheism to my kids. I engage in discussions with them about religion, and I've told them that I believe that Grandma and Granddad are looking down at them from Heaven.

But I know I'll never look down on them that way. And that hurts.

I've just read back over this post so far. Man, it's dark. Quite a difference after two days of funny hat pictures. Sorry about that.

Looking back, I think I knew I was teetering on the edge of a black hole and I probably tried my best to sound cheerful.

I could do that now; pretend that everything is hunky dory - but that's not what this blog is about. I promised I would be 100% open and honest, and that's what I'm trying to do.

Cancer plus depression does not equal happy Tommy.

Please understand - I'm not trying to make you feel sorry for me. If it was up to me, I'd probably just stay in bed and not post anything today.

But I started this blog to chart my battle against this disease, and that means writing on the bad days as well as the good.

I know it could be worse. I know they've caught the cancer in time to treat it, at least for now.

I know it's not going to kill me. Yet.

And that scares me, too.

How stupid does that sound?

I know I'm going to be ill. Very ill. But I'll still have to find a way to provide for my family. I'm terrified I'm going to let them down, more than I already have.

There - that's the depression talking again. Bastard.

I'd better sign off now before you all click away and never come back. I'll try to make tomorrow's update a little more positive.

If I can.

TO SLEEP, PERCHANCE...

"**M**idnight," as the great *Shakin' Stevens* once sang, "one more night without sleeping..."

He knew what he was talking about, did Shaky.

I'm doing it again. Sitting up at my desk, wide awake, while the rest of the family sleep. I tried to nod off a few times earlier, but couldn't settle and so I got up again.

I'm really nervous about tomorrow. Well, today now. More specifically, my 2pm appointment with the radiographer to discuss my treatment.

That sounds ridiculous, doesn't it? These people have come up with a plan of action to rid me of cancer, and I'm scared to go and hear what they have to say.

I think it's the unknown. I know nothing about chemotherapy, or radiotherapy and quite frankly I'm too much of a coward to look up the details online. I just know I'll come across some little detail or glance at some horrible image that will have me crapping myself.

Look at me - the big man who can't even look at pictures

of his own disease. How am I supposed to beat this thing if I'm too scared to face it, eye to eye?

Jesus, that sent a shiver up my spine. I hope it hasn't got eyes!

So, here I am. Sitting at my desk in the middle of the night, reading web forums I never usually get around to visiting. I suppose that's something, at least.

The doctor gave me some sleeping tablets. I'm going to take a couple soon, and head back to bed for another attempt at visiting the land of nod.

Did you know that The Land of Nod is mentioned in the Bible? It's in Genesis, and is reported to be to the east of the Garden of Eden. That's my favourite pub quiz question ever.

East of Eden. My sister, Sue, loves that film, along with anything else to do with James Dean.

When you're brought up Catholic, you get 'confirmed' as a teenager and have to choose an extra name. A confirmation name. It's supposed to be a religious name that means something important to you. The name of someone from religious history you have researched and, as a result, admire.

Sue chose the name Caleb because that's the character James Dean played in East of Eden! She got away with it, too.

I chose Matthew, because he was a writer.

For someone who doesn't believe in God, he's been on my mind a lot lately. I've had messages from so many people saying that they are praying for me. It's very humbling, and I'm trying to reply to them all to say thank you.

Earlier this evening, my 9 year old son, Sam, asked me what I would ask for if I was granted three wishes. I told him to go first.

He said he'd ask for...

- A cure for cancer
- World peace

- Twelve more genies (because you can't wish for more wishes)

He's amazing. Both my boys are. I love them so much, and I know they're going to be scared and upset as they watch me go through my treatment.

And there's nothing I can do about it.

I don't think I've ever felt more helpless than I have done over the past two weeks. Since I got my diagnosis. There's literally nothing I can do to get over this other than submit to weeks of chemical and radioactive bombardment.

And I'm too scared to find out more about either.

Cancer sucks.

A MAN WITH A PLAN

O K, doc... Give it to me straight!"
Alright, I didn't say it quite like that - but I did ask the consultant radiologist at Blackburn Hospital to be honest with me during our meeting to discuss my cancer treatment this afternoon.

He certainly did that. And then some.

My treatment will most likely begin the week after next, when I will have to attend five radiotherapy sessions per week - Monday to Friday - at Royal Preston Hospital. On one of those days - most likely Wednesday - I'll be treated with chemotherapy as well.

It's an all-out attack on the cancer in my system.

But, there are one or two things that need to be done first...

I had dental x-rays taken at the hospital last week and, today, I saw the ENT department's resident dental surgeon for a check-up. He explained that radiotherapy can and will attack the teeth of cancer patients - although no-one knows exactly why.

The challenge is to identify any weaknesses in the teeth

before treatment begins to minimise complications after-wards. The result - I've got one dodgy tooth that will be removed next week.

I also have two baby teeth left with no adult versions queued up behind them, but they're staying for the time being.

The dentist went into a lot of detail. He told me that the radiotherapy will effectively kill my lower jaw, but that it will take years to die. As a result, I may suffer from dental prob-lems for the rest of my life.

There's a happy thought.

I also have to have a metal cage/mask moulded to fit my head before I can have my radiotherapy. They showed me a sample. At first, I hoped I was being fitted for some kind of titanium body armour (well, normal guy plus radio waves does equal superhero), but that doesn't seem to be the case.

I also have to have a feeding tube inserted through my skin and directly into my stomach. The reason, because it won't be too long before I can't drink, chew or swallow. So, I'll need to be fed liquids through my tube.

Oh boy.

"You're going to be ill," the consultant told me. "Very ill." In fact, he went on to say that, no matter how bleak and horrible he makes this sound, it's going to be at least a hundred times worse.

Here are a few highlights...

- You'll feel like you've got sunburn on the inside.
- The outside of your neck will burn and blister.
- After a week or two, you won't be able to drive.
- Or work.
- Or talk.

"If there was any alternative to what you're about to go

through," he said, "I would urge you to take it. I would tell you to run now, and not look back."

"But, there isn't an alternative. You have to go through this."

I have to admit - I like him.

But, wow...

Would anyone mind if I crapped my pants?

Six weeks of radio and chemo, followed by at least a three month recuperation period. Then speech therapy and further dental work, if necessary.

There goes 2016.

HEEEEERE'S BARRY!

H*ello!*

I'm Barry, a friend of Tommy's. He's roped me in to help run the site should he ever find himself too unwell to post an update. I'm interrupting his banging on about illness and hospitals an' that to post this. Don't tell him.

Tommy and I first met online via a writer's website about 15 years ago. We hit it off right away, sharing a similar sense of humour and the same drive to become full-time writers.

Over the years, our careers have strangely mirrored one another. Tommy started writing his spooky children's series, *Scream Street*, and soon after that my own horror series was picked up.

I wrote some stuff for the telly, then around the same time Tommy started writing for the TV version of his *Scream Street* series.

We both write for *The Beano*, constantly swap ideas, and have run joint events in schools to promote our love of reading and writing. I was even the best man at Tommy's wedding, where I took immense pleasure in heavily promoting my books throughout my speech.

I talk to Tommy every day via Skype. For a decade and a half he has been my constant companion as I've tried to navigate my way through the topsy-turvy world of children's publishing.

And he has cancer.

I knew Tommy hadn't been well. I knew he had an appointment to get a worrying lump on his throat checked, but I reassured him that it'd be fine. Nothing to worry about. One of those things.

Only, it wasn't.

Tommy told me about his diagnosis shortly after getting home from the hospital. For the first time in 15 years, I didn't know what to say. We've both discussed the illness itself several times over the years — both Tommy's parents and my mum succumbed to it — but this was different. I just stared at the words he had written on screen, hoping I'd somehow misread them, or misunderstood their meaning.

I can't remember what I finally did say. I swore, I think. Nothing particularly helpful, anyway. Tommy, however, said two things which I think go some way to reveal the man he is. He said:

"I feel like I've let Kirsty (his wife) and the kids down."

and:

"I'm glad my mum and dad aren't here to worry about me."

Those were his first thoughts. Not, "why me?" or "it's not fair" or "how am I going to cope?" His first thoughts were for those around him, and how it was going to affect them.

And that's Tommy. That's why I've spoken to him on a daily basis for 15 years. That's why other authors — some who have never even met him — have been contacting me asking what they can do to help.

Like myself and most children's authors, the majority of Tommy's income doesn't actually come from writing at all. It comes from speaking events at schools, festivals and libraries. This horrible illness has taken those speaking opportunities away from Tommy, leaving an enormous hole in his finances.

Sadly, the world doesn't care about any of that. The bills will keep coming, demanding to be paid, and so Tommy has had to find a way to generate a new source of income, so he can continue to provide for his family.

Tommy has spent the last 7 years travelling around the UK teaching children and adults how to write fantastic stories, and he's now making all that knowledge available via Patreon.com. From as little as $1 (about 70p) a month, you can become a Patron, and sponsor Tommy to create exclusive video and written content on the subject of creative writing.

Tommy doesn't like talking about his Patreon, as he hates the idea of asking people for money. I'm more than happy to talk about it, though, because he isn't asking for money at all – he's offering you the bargain of a lifetime.

In just a few years, Tommy has written almost 100 books as well as TV scripts, comic strips and pretty much any other type of creative writing you can think of. He has delivered workshops to thousands of children and adults, and I can think of no-one better placed to give advice to aspiring writers of all ages. What's more, Patrons will also be helping ensure Tommy can continue to writes the type of stories which turn reluctant readers into lifelong book-lovers. That's got to be worth a few quid a month in anyone's book.

We can't fight Tommy's cancer for him, but we can buy him the time he needs to fight it himself. It's a one-on-one fight to the finish – Tommy V Cancer – but by God, I'm honoured to be standing there in his corner holding his towel. I hope you'll join me there.

To find out more, visit:

www.patreon.com/tommydonbavand

Cheers,

Barry

PS - Tommy mentioned in an earlier post that once his hair goes he won't be able to wear a woolly hat, as he says they make him look like a serial killer. I told him he was being silly. Then he sent me a photo of how he looks in one.

He's right. He must never be allowed to wear a woolly hat.

THE GORY DETAILS

Yesterday I spent the afternoon at the hospital, chatting with Sharron - the Macmillan head and neck cancer nurse - and Lucy, my new speech therapist. They took me through my forthcoming treatment in great detail, answering all my questions, and preparing me for what is to come.

The biggest shock came when Sharron explained why they aren't attempting to operate to remove the cancer. Essentially, it's inoperable. Because of where they cancer is, and how it has spread - if they were to operate, they would have to remove my entire tongue, and a lot of the soft tissue inside my mouth.

This would leave me unable to talk ever again. And I would have to be fed through a stomach tube permanently.

Wow.

So, they're giving my cancer both barrels with the radio and chemotherapy in the hope that will be enough to eradicate it.

Fingers crossed.

They took me through how my mask will be moulded to

my face, and used to keep me perfectly still while I'm being bombarded by the radiation.

Things aren't looking too good for my salivary glands and the skin of my neck and throat - which are essentially going to fry. They asked if I wanted to see photographs of what that will look like.

I politely declined.

They explained how my stomach feeding tube - or 'peg' - will be fitted next week, and how I will eventually be unable to eat and have to feed myself with nutrient packed milk through it.

Can't say I'm looking forward to that.

Although that's when I'm most likely to lose weight - which can only be a good thing. I often wonder whether the cancer would be so bad, or even if it would be there at all, if I'd taken better care of myself over the years.

Too late to think like that now.

When my throat is frazzled and I can no longer produce much, if any, saliva, my vocal chords are going to suffer. Hence the need for Lucy, the speech and swallow therapist. She said it's quite possible my voice may be different when it eventually returns.

That will be weird. I wonder what - or who - I'll sound like? It's as though this cancer is robbing me of, well... me.

Bit by bit. Piece by piece.

My chemotherapy sessions - one per week - will last for five hours at a time. I've been advised to bring a book!

Still, the good news there is that this particular dose of chemo means I won't lose my hair!

Well, there's a silver lining.

I'll also be given an emergency telephone number to use should I develop any kind of illness or temperature during my treatment. Even something as simple as a stomach bug or heavy cold could have major consequences if my ability to fight the infection has been reduced.

That would mean being admitted to hospital straight away, hence the 24 hour emergency telephone number. Under no circumstances am I to wait and see how I feel in the morning.

Wow. Again.

This is far more complicated than I could ever have imagined. I have stacks and stacks of reading material to get through, each leaflet and letter providing yet more detail of the horrors I'm about to face.

I don't want this. At all.

I don't want to be strapped to a table by a head mask while being targeted by radio waves.

I don't want chemicals pumped into my system once a week.

I don't want to lose the ability to speak and eat.

I don't want to have to feed myself through a tube that runs directly into my stomach.

I don't want to have cancer.

SLEEPING UGLY

It's now 3.19am.

Another sleepless night.

I gave up trying to read about an hour ago and now, here I am, sitting at my desk again.

The lump has been really hurting today. I had plans to crack on with my work-in-progress - the first book in a new series I'm writing for *Oxford University Press* - but I just couldn't concentrate through the pain.

Kirsty had to get the morphine and help me into bed for a while.

That's a bit of a worry.

The publishers have already extended my deadline to help me with my current situation, and I don't want to miss the new date if I can avoid doing so.

I should launch the file and get a few hundred words written now, seeing as I'm not busy with anything else, but I don't want to really wake myself up and still be sitting here at dawn.

My body clock is suffering enough without me switching daytime for night-time.

So, I'm browsing websites and reading blogs. A less important, but easier to handle use of my time.

I sometimes wonder if I should watch a movie when I'm awake like this, you know - headphones plugged into the iPad. But, the truth is, I don't want to do anything. I just want the time to pass, and for it to be morning again.

It's Easter Sunday tomorrow. Well, today. Kirsty and the boys have a nice little pile of chocolate eggs to get through (knowing the boys, from the moment they wake up!)

In a way, I hope they do. Sam (9) has hardly been eating since he found out about my cancer and treatment. He leaves meals half-finished, or more. He avoids snacks. He barely touches his breakfast before school.

I'm worried about him, but don't want to tell him off for leaving food because I know why he's doing it.

Sam suffers from Asperger's Syndrome, and all that comes along with that diagnosis. He's very high-functioning, knows everything about his chosen subject (penguins!), and he's already decided that he wants to work with the birds when he's older.

We were watching TV one day (a documentary about penguins, as you might suspect) when a guy came on screen. The info on the bottom of the picture announced him as a 'penguinologist', to which Sam cried - that's what I want to be!

Several hours of online research later, he knew that he would need to do well in his GCSEs at school, take certain 'A' levels at college, and then study marine biology at university before specialising in penguins.

But, the payoff to this intelligence is a fear of change. He likes and frequently needs things to stay the same in order for him to be able to process them - and my cancer is about as big a change as I can imagine.

He asked to see my stomach tube today, saying that he

knew it was called a 'peg'. I explained that I don't have it fitted until next week. He was a little shaken, and said that he had dreamed I'd already had it put in place.

So, he's dreaming about my treatment. Just like me, when I can sleep, that is. No wonder he's lost his appetite. I hope he can forget that for one day and just get stuck into his Easter eggs.

The same for Kirsty and Arran.

No eggs for me though - which isn't a form of self-denial or anything. I just don't like chocolate. Or sweets. Or crisps. Or cakes. Or ice cream. Or desserts.

I have the opposite of a sweet tooth. Always have.

I'm a weirdo.

The dental consultant said it was clear from my x-ray that I don't have a sweet tooth - otherwise those on the screen would be in a worse state of disrepair.

So, that's something.

Taste buds renew themselves every ten days. Did you know that? I found out as part of the research I did for an article I wrote in Amazing! magazine a few months back.

Mine are about to be nuked for six weeks straight.

The nurse said that, when they finally grow back, I may find that I have different tastes. I may like and dislike different foods compared to know.

I might get a sweet tooth!

Damn, I hope not.

I've managed to get as overweight as I am now without the help of sugary treats, crisps, cakes and sticky desserts.

I don't need any help in that direction.

Still, I'll soon have my stomach tube to help me lose a few pounds. The nurse warned me that some patients get addicted to losing weight via the peg and don't go back to eating the natural way when th-

Whoah.

It's now - quarter past four. Thirty five minutes later. I just dozed off, at my desk, while writing a blog post. Right in the middle of a sentence. Then... WHAM! Awake with a start, no idea where I am.

I really can't go on like this.

BRING IT ON!

J ust a quick update today as I've spent most of the day in bed - this time due to pain, rather than being depressed. But, the end result is much the same.

I've just got up to have something to eat (soup, as usual!), then I'm heading back to bed to read for a while and - hopefully - get some sleep.

I want this pain to be over. I want the cancer to go away. And, as there's only one way that's going to happen, I wonder if I'm starting to be keen for the therapy to begin?

I never thought I'd hear myself say this but, yes - bring it on. Let's get this party started!

The messages of support continue to flood in from all over the world, and I'm very grateful for each and everyone one of them.

I'll try to reply to everyone individually but, if I can't, please be aware that I read every email, tweet or dm, and that they all help me stay positive in the face of the fight.

Thank you.

THE WHOLE TOOTH

U p early this morning to get a bit of writing done before I have to head back to Blackburn Hospital - to have a tooth removed.

Apparently, radiotherapy can cause problems for any weak teeth, or those with existing problems (although nobody knows exactly how or why), so it's common for the ENT department's resident dental surgeon to remove any suspect teeth before treatment starts.

The tooth I'm having removed today is one which received extensive root canal work back in the late 90s. I remember the situation well. Not only did the treatment last for several sessions (and was, therefore, very expensive), but my dentist at the time strongly resembled an Indian Robin Williams.

Somehow that made all the painful drilling that little bit easier.

The dentist I'll be seeing today doesn't look like anyone famous (or at least, no-one that I know). But he was very open and honest about the way my forthcoming radiotherapy is going to essentially kill my lower jaw - but that it will take years to die.

He also pointed out two baby teeth on my dental x-ray which have remained in place because I had no adult teeth waiting beneath them. That's three baby teeth in all, as Robin Williams had to remove one of those 20-something years ago, too.

After my appointment, I'll be heading back to my desk to crack on with work. I want to try to get as much writing done as possible before I feel either too ill, too tired, or I'm in too much pain to sit at my desk for any worthwhile period of time.

UPDATE: My appointment had to be postponed at the last minute as my mouth was too swollen and sore for the tooth to be removed. It's now all happening this Sunday, 3rd April, at 7am!

MUM

In December, 2005, my Mum - Elizabeth Mary Donbavand - died. And I was there when it happened.

She had cancer, and so it's no surprise that I've been thinking about her a lot over the past week or two. My Dad, too - although I'm going to write about him in a separate post.

My Mum hadn't been well for a long time and, if she was honest, she knew what the problem was. She had breathing problems, a hacking cough, and she was in constant pain.

But she didn't want anyone to tell her what the diagnosis was. She didn't want to hear anyone say that word.

So, she struggled on for several years, becoming more and more unwell, refusing to go to the doctor, and self-medicating for the agonising pain.

Don't get me wrong - we all tried to convince her that she should get treatment, but she was a stubborn so-and-so, my mum. In the end, all we could do was respect her wishes, and help care for her as best we could.

In 2005, I was living in a town called Bedlington in the north east of England - around 10 miles north of Newcastle. I was working for a children's theatre company, and I had recently met Kirsty - the girl who would later become my wife.

Then, at 5.40am on 28th November, my mobile 'phone rang.

How can I be so sure of the exact time and date? 28th November is my birthday, and my Mum always told me that I'd been born at 5.40am. At first, I thought someone was playing a joke by calling to wish me a happy birthday at the exact moment of my arrival into the world.

I couldn't have been more wrong.

The 'phone call was from my brother, Bryan. He told me that Mum had been taken into hospital by ambulance a few hours earlier, and things didn't look good.

I didn't know what to do, so I asked him to call back if there were any further developments. He promised that he would.

He rang again 20 minutes later, saying he thought I had better get there as quickly as I could.

I was 160 miles away.

At that time, my car was off the road, and so I was using one of the theatre company's large touring vans to get around. It was currently parked outside the house. I tried to call my bosses to get their permission to use the van, with no luck (it was still the early hours of the morning), so I just decided to take it.

Kirsty and I set off on the 160 mile drive to Chorley in Lancashire, where I knew my Mum was now being moved into the intensive care unit. It was a tough drive, especially as I didn't know what I would be faced with when I got there.

By the time we got to the hospital, my entire family was already in the ICU waiting room: my Dad, brother, sister and my mum's brother and sister. The doctors were making some adjustments to my Mum's treatments on the ward, so I had to wait 40 minutes before could I go in and see her.

Then, I was told I wouldn't be able to talk with her.

In order to keep her stable, the doctors had put her into a medically induced coma. She was unconscious. She wouldn't even know that I was there.

A very long 40 minutes later, I was allowed in. My Dad came with me. It was a shock, seeing my Mum lying in this huge hospital bed, attached to drips, a feeding tubes, oxygen, etc.

She looked so small.

I stood at the side of the bed and said, "You know, there are easier ways to get to see me on my birthday!"

Suddenly, my Mum - deep in her coma - started moving around, waving her arms and kicking her legs. It set off alarms on several of her monitors. All at the sound of my voice.

She knew I was there.

For the next week, we sat at my Mum's bedside, holding her hand and chatting to her. She didn't move or react again.

Hours were spent, sitting in the tiny family waiting room beside the unit. We were only allowed on the ward in groups of two or three at a time so, whenever friends or other family members arrived, I'd wait out in the family room. I bought puzzle book after puzzle book at the hospital shop, and completed them all.

Then, towards the end of the week, the doctors gathered us together and said they were going to try to put a stent in my Mum's throat; a small mesh tube that would allow her to breathe on her own. That would mean she could come home for however long she had left, and be with the family for the end.

But that meant waking her up. That meant she would know what was going on.

That meant they would tell her she had cancer. She would know she was about to die.

And she would be very, very scared.

So, after a long conversation, we decided against the stent. We all agreed that it would be better for my Mum if we were to let her slip away without waking up. Without ever having to hear that word.

Without knowing she was about to die.

Everything happened very quickly after that. We had gone to the hospital cafe for a break when a nurse rushed in to call us back to the ICU.

This was it.

I ran outside to get my sister, who was making a 'phone call, and we gathered together around my Mum's bed. The nurses drew the curtains around us.

I was terrified. Partly because I suddenly realised that I had never seen a dead body before, and the first one I was going to see would be my Mum's.

But, mainly because of the machines she was hooked up to. I knew the readings were going to fall steadily until they reached zero. And I didn't want to hear that sound. I didn't want to hear the flat line.

We took turns holding her hand, telling her how much we loved her, and assuring her that everyone was safe and that she didn't need to worry about us.

We told her that her much-missed Mum (my Nan) was waiting for her, along with all her other Irish relatives, and that she would be drinking endless cups of tea and gossiping with them all again in no time.

All she had to do was let go.

And, eventually, she did. She took one last, deep breath, and left this world.

Out of the corner of my eye, through my tears, I saw a

nurse's hand quickly reach through the curtain to silence the machines. They knew how scared I was of hearing them.

They asked us to step out for 20 minutes and, when we returned, the monitors and tubes were all gone. My Mum was dressed in a white gown, and she looked as though she was in a deep, peaceful sleep. Beside her was a silver tray on which sat a copy of The Bible and a white flower.

Before we left, the nurses gave us each a card containing a poem about how death was never the end. Clipped inside each one was a lock of my Mum's hair.

My Mum - Elizabeth Mary Donbavand - was the strongest, bravest, most amazing woman I have ever met, and could have ever had as a Mum. She was 59 years old when she died. Just 11 years older than I am now.

Once, when I was first starting out as an entertainer, she sat up all night, hand-sewing sequins on to the jacket of my clown costume.

When I was in the musical *Buddy*, she always waved to me from the audience at the start of the show, even though she knew I couldn't wave back.

One day, when we were shopping together, she saw a doormat that read 'Wipe your feet, stupid!', and she laughed so much it nearly made her sick.

As the doctors put her into her coma at the hospital - while I was driving to get to her bedside - my Mum, who could no longer talk, pointed to my Dad, touched her wedding ring, and then touched her heart.

She told him that she had loved being married to him.

God, I wish she was here to help me through this now.

PEG IT

Back from an overnight stay in hospital, where I had a feeding tube or 'peg' fitted. This tube will allow me to consume nutrient rich milkshakes, should I become utterly unable to eat or drink during my periods of radiotherapy and chemotherapy.

I have to admit to being very nervous when I arrived on the ward, not least because the first thing the nurses did was hook me up to a drip filled with antibiotics.

What kind of procedure is so nasty that it comes with medicine in advance?

This one. This one does.

Once I'd taken the antibiotics on board, I was wheeled down to the operating theatre where I was gleefully informed that my peg would be fitted under local anaesthetic, and that I would be awake the whole time.

Can you imagine the fun I was having by this point.

It got funnier.

No, really.

I had to lie back on the table while I had another drip fitted

- this one full of sedatives - and the back of my throat was sprayed. Then the nurse produced an endoscope (one of those cameras that goes down your throat and into your stomach).

You see, everyone's stomach is in a slightly different position - so they have to look inside in order to be able to accurately pinpoint it. It turns out that, because of a liver operation I had as a toddler, my stomach sits quite high in my body.

So, camera in - blowing air to allow access on the way down and into my stomach, where they switched on a bright light fixed to the end. That shone through my skin, showing the surgeon exactly where to cut.

And cut, he did.

Then, he produced a length of wire, which he inserted through the hole, into my stomach and over the head of the endoscope. The endoscope was then removed bringing the wire with it.

The camera came out, and I was now essentially threaded with one end of the wire jutting from my mouth, and the other from a hole in my stomach.

"This next bit isn't going to be very pleasant," said a nurse.

Hahahaha! This next bit!

Dear God, she was right!

The nurse attached one end of my peg (the feeding tube) to the wire sticking out of my mouth, and then the surgeon pulled hard on the other end.

With a sound I can only describe at GASCHLOINK!, the peg slid down my throat, through my upper body and emerged glistening out of my stomach.

They fitted my feeding tube into my stomach via my mouth!

A few adjustments later, and I was done. I spent 20

minutes or so in the recovery room, then wheeled back up to the ward.

But, the fun wasn't over quite yet...

I hadn't been able to eat or drink since 8am, and it was now 3pm. To say I was peckish was something of an under-statement.

"You can have something to eat once we're sure the peg has taken," explained one of the nurses. "It should only take six hours or so."

Yep. I lay in that bed with a throat like a sandy flip flop for another six hours.

Then, at 9pm, a doctor came along to test the peg.

Attaching a large syringe to the free end, he proceeded to pour 50ml of water into the gizmo which - thanks purely to effects of gravity - vanished straight into my stomach.

It was the weirdest sensation of my life!

But, it worked! They said I could eat again!

They brought me a mug of Bovril.

"No solids until the morning!"

sob

Mind you, that was the most amazing mug of Bovril I'd ever had, second only to the second mug one of the nurses quietly slipped me an hour later when the doctor wasn't looking!

So, that's me with a peg fitted.

UPDATE: Before I was allowed home today, I was given some training on how to feed myself through the peg, should I become unable to eat or drink during my therapy.

One of the very important things I have to do is rinse it through with water once a day, just to make sure it's running freely.

So, when I got home, I unclipped the end of the peg, attached the syringe and poured in 50ml of water.

Thanks to gravity, all went well for the first 30ml.

Then the liquid bubbled slightly...

...and the bastard started to run backwards!

The syringe was quickly filling up with horrible, semi-digested bits of Weetabix (my solid treat at breakfast), presumably swimming in my own, personal brand of digestive juices!

I screamed and quickly pushed the cap back in place.

I thought I was about to turn inside out. Or, at the very least, act like one of those old vacuum cleaners in comics; the ones that you could switch from 'suck' to 'blow'.

All I could picture was my utterly deflated body lying in a room where everything was slowly dissolving around me!

One hasty 'phone call to the hospital later, I was advised that I probably still had air in my stomach from the endoscopy yesterday. They said they probably should have warned me about that.

Yes, I think they probably should.

OUCHY!

I t's 3am, and all's well...

Actually, no it's not. I can't sleep because of the pain.

Again.

But then, someone did dig a hole through my skin and into one of my internal organs yesterday, so perhaps that's not surprising.

Plus, it's made me forget about the pain of the lump in my throat for a while.

Hooray.

I really must try to get some sleep. I have to crack on with work again from tomorrow. My editor for the new series has very kindly extended my deadline for the first draft of the first book by another week, which is a huge help.

Still, that means writing a couple of thousand words per day - every day - for the next ten days to meet that date.

It's doable, but it will be tough. I'm terrified they'll decide to cancel the series and demand the advance back. That'll be me shafted if that happens.

I don't like missing deadlines. I always try to get my

books in on time, or early if possible. I just haven't had the energy - or peace of mind - to sit at my desk for long periods of time lately.

I also have two reluctant readers shorts to write this weekend. They will be books 93 and 94 in my catalogue. Nearly at 100...

I'm allowed a day off when I hit 100 books. ;)

Ow!

There's just no way to sit with this thing that's comfortable. Although I did manage to flush it properly before bed. And by 'properly', I mean without the horror movie special effects and the sound of me screaming like a four year old girl.

The specialist peg nurse (yes) said that the first 72 hours are crucial and that if anything goes wrong with the peg during that time I'm to call an ambulance or get to A&E immediately.

Maybe that's another reason why I'm not sleeping.

I should have been visiting a primary school yesterday. And, not just any primary school - the school where my cousin's three daughters go. I was really looking forward to it.

I had to cancel the visit, for obvious reasons.

I've had to cancel a lot of school visits. Festival appearances, too. Including my first invitation to appear at the *Bath Children's Literature Festival*. I'm hoping they'll have me back.

Everyone has been incredibly understanding when I've explained that I'm having to cancel due to my health. Well, almost everyone...

I received an email from a teacher saying that one of his pupils was devastated that I had cancelled my visit, and was now in constant tears. He'd brought his entire collection of *Scream Street* books in for me to sign, and I hadn't shown up.

In fact, when he'd told his class that I was wasn't coming because I was unwell, they'd looked at him as if he'd "just shot a puppy".

Great.

To be fair, he did offer his good wishes when I replied to explain just what kind of unwell I was. And I emailed the boy a set of signed bookplates to say sorry.

I hate letting people down, but there's nothing I can do.

I'd much rather not have cancer and be able to meet my readers.

I really can't express just how wonderful everyone has been. And helpful. And caring. And generous. And loving.

And more.

Part of me thinks I really don't deserve all that affection. There are so many people with far more serious illnesses than me – you just don't hear about them because they aren't narcissistic enough to blog about every tiny detail.

But, I know that's the depression again, lurking at the back of my mind. I have to be careful not to let that bugger out of its cage. It would have a field day with this peg situation.

Bloody peg.

I'll be getting boxes of nutrient milkshakes delivered directly to my door every month. In a range of flavours.

Yes, flavours.

Apparently you can drink them as well as stuff them down the tube.

Who knew?

Kirsty made a fantastic lasagne tonight. It was really soft, so even I could eat it without too much throat pain. Although when she served it up, Sam sat and scowled at it for a while before asking how I was going to get it through my peg.

I explained that not everything has to go down that way. Well, not yet anyway.

We decided that if I did have to eat pasta that way, then it would have to be single strands of spaghetti, but the meat-balls might prove to be a bit of a problem.

I'm really worried about Sam. He's still being very quiet, and not eating properly. And he's vomited once or twice over the past few days for no discernible reason.

He's not coping very well with all this.

I didn't know what his reaction would be when I showed him the peg. So, we stopped at the hospital shop on the way out and picked him up a present - a teddy version of the baby hare from Sam McBratney's amazing book, *Guess How Much I Love You*.

He loved it.

Then I asked if he was ready to see the peg, claiming that this latest addition officially made me Dad 2.0...

He looked at it for a second, then said, "Is that it?"

I don't know what he was expecting.

But then, I know he's very much like me. He'll build things up in his mind until they're much bigger and far more terrifying than they could ever be in real life.

I hope he'll be OK.

I mustn't forget about Arran, either. He may be big and tall and all teenagery now, but that doesn't mean he isn't also my son. My little boy. I still worry about him, too.

I just don't think he'd appreciate a teddy bear.

He's coping by not talking about my situation at all, and that's fine by me. So long as he knows that I'll still be here if and when he changes his mind about that.

3.30am and all's well.

Ish.

Ow.

I'M A TROLL, FOL-DE-ROL

I had a strange experience over the weekend: the first negative response to my public fight against cancer.

I don't want to give the guy any further oxygen of publicity, so I won't name him here. Instead, for the purposes of this blog post, I'll call him Troll (you have NO idea how many names I typed and deleted just then!)

In order to attract attention to my blog, I tweeted a handful of people I admire and asked if they would be kind enough to re-tweet the link to where I write about my battle with cancer.

The brilliant Reverend Richard Coles (formerly of The Communards, now a popular support act for God) did just that. I got a lot of new visitors as a result.

Then, a message popped up on Twitter...

TROLL: Why do people battle cancer? Do they battle heart disease? I've had cancer. You take the medicine - battle?

I have to admit, it took me a little by surprise. I don't know this guy, so why does it matter to him what I call how I deal with my illness.

So, I tweeted back...

ME: To me and my young family it is, yes.

And from there, the conversation went like this...

TROLL: I took the surgery, chemo, radio - I did not "battle".

ME: I'm delighted to hear it. I, however, choose to battle.

TROLL: I wish you well but how does the battle manifest itself other than you taking the medicine?

ME: Mental attitude, staying positive for my two scared sons, and more. Thanks for the advice, however.

TROLL: Of course that's important but it is the treatment that does the main work.

ME: I understand the process, thank you.

At this point, I decided that there was nothing to be gained by engaging with this person, and so ignored him.

However, my sister, Sue, was not impressed by his comments, and told him so...

SUE: Thanks for taking the time to belittle how my brother chooses to address HIS illness, note the emphasis on his, not yours.

TROLL: I think you will find my comments were generic rather than personal.

SUE: You made it personal by taking it upon yourself to question him. If he feels like it's a battle, then it's a battle.

TROLL: I think if you read carefully I was not questioning him but the specific concept of battle.

SUE: Then maybe address them to generic people, not in response to someone just diagnosed with cancer?

TROLL: I wish your brother well: but a blog is a public forum and I, who had surgery, chemo and radio am also entitled to my opinion.

SUE: It's your right to call however you deal with your own illness whatever you want, his to do the same. Good night.

TROLL: Did I suggest otherwise? Many on Twitter seem to 2nd guess.

SUE: Well, each to their own. I get no pleasure from making a man, newly diagnosed with a scary illness, explain himself.

TROLL: If you read my tweets you will see none is personal.

SUE: If that makes you feel better, you think like that. Goodnight.

And on the conversation went on...

...and continued the next day with my very good friend, Barry Hutchison...

BARRY: The willingness to go through great hardship in the hope of staying alive is a very clear definition of "battling" IMO. I am perplexed why you'd feel the need to chime in on the statement, frankly.

TROLL: Because when I had cancer there was no battle - I let the surgery, chemo & radio do their work. Battle is tabloid speak.

BARRY: But my point is, why question how someone describes their situation? Positive mind-set and drive to beat illness can only help.

TROLL: My question was generic rather than personal - I am not familiar with survival data on positive mind - I doubt major effect.

BARRY: You say it was a generic remark, but you made it direct to someone making a personal statement about their own illness.

TROLL: True but in a public forum.

BARRY: So make your generic comments in a public forum, but not aimed at someone in particular. Did he aim his tweet at you directly?

TROLL: It came via a RT but a blog is intended as a public forum - surely?

BARRY: Forget it. Life's too short to discuss this any further with you. Like I say, though... If, on hearing a person has cancer, my first instinct would not be to question the words they chose to describe their situation.

TROLL: I was not questioning that but asking why? There is a difference.

And on the thread went, round and round, until Barry very wisely gave up.

Basically, this clown was saying to me...

"You're doing cancer wrong! Do it my way!"

Er... no thanks, fella. I'll decide what I decide to call the way I face my illness. If I decide it's a battle, then it's a battle. And it's got sod all to do with you.

I have to admit to expecting one or two negative comments about the very public way in which I'm charting my fight against this terrible disease. And I'm not in the slightest bit bothered by what this guy had to say.

The messages of support, love, prayers, help and good vibes that I receive every day FAR outweigh anything a mere Twitter troll could try to impose on my outlook.

So [NAME REDACTED] - go and boil your head!

And that sentence needed rewriting a few times, too!

TAKE A LETTER

I received a 'phone call this afternoon from the cancer centre at the Royal Preston Hospital. It went something like this...

RPH: Is there any reason you didn't attend your planning appointment with us this morning?

ME: Er... Because no-one told me I had a planning appointment.

RPH: Yes, we did. We sent you a letter.

ME: Nope, didn't get that.

RPH: Really? What's your address?

ME: It's this [*gives address*]

RPH: Ah!

ME: What?

RPH: We've got the wrong address.

ME: Oh. Which address do you have?

RPH: This... [*reads out address*]

ME: What?! That was the house I grew up in. I haven't lived there for over 30 years. My Dad sold that house 10 years ago after my Mum died.

RPH: Oh. Where did we get that, then?

ME: I've no idea!

RPH: Give me your correct address again.

ME: Sure, it's this... [*gives address again*]

RPH: Can you come in tomorrow?

ME: Yes, no problem.

RPH: Great! Your radiotherapy treatment begins two weeks today - on Monday 18th April.

CLICK

So, I have a date for my treatment to start.

Monday 18th April 2016.

In Preston.

I really hope they can target high-energy x-rays better than they can letters...

ON THE STAGE

At my request, I wasn't told what type of cancer I have, or at what stage it was when I was first diagnosed. I simply didn't want that stuff playing on my mind.

However, as Kirsty and I have come to fill in paperwork for PIP funding and other available benefits, the forms have asked for detailed information.

And so, I had to email my Macmillan nurse for the details.

She got back to me this evening.

Ready? I have Squamous cell carcinoma right tonsil and tongue base T4 N2b M0.

T4 N2b M0.

Individually, those codes are reasonably innocent...

T4 refers to the size and spread of the original cancer, and that it is present in my tissue and bones.

N2b means it has spread to two lymph nodes, up to a size of 6cm.

M0 says it hasn't spread to my lungs, brain or other vital organs.

Together, they mean I have stage four cancer.

The worst it can possibly be.

The news has hit me hard. Just when I thought there was nothing else that could land a punch.

This is why my cancer is inoperable.

Or at least - inoperable without removing my tongue and a good portion of my inner mouth. That would render me unable to talk or eat naturally.

I spent a lot of time crying tonight while Kirsty held me.

I don't want this. I don't want this for me, or my family.

Obviously, I haven't told the boys. They're scared enough as it is.

Sam gave me a cuddle earlier and he accidentally pressed his hand against my stomach peg. I winced in pain, and he ended up in tears.

He thought he'd really hurt me.

I had to pretend he hadn't.

The head teacher at his school is concerned for him, and pulled him out of class for a chat today to see how he's been getting on.

They're prepared to arrange counselling for him if it's required.

I was visited by the district nurse today, who offered the same thing for him....

"Someone can come out from the local hospice and talk to him."

No, no, no. Please, please don't let him hear the word 'hospice'. He may only be 9 years old, but he's smart. He knows exactly what a hospice is for.

If he hears that word, he'll jump to all the wrong conclusions.

She offered me counselling, too.

I said I wasn't sure. That I'd think about it.

I'm still thinking.

Would a counsellor help me? Do I have the same thoughts as everyone else who goes through this shit?

What, when it comes down to it, am I worried about?

I'm forcing myself to think here...

I'm not worried about dying. At least, I don't think so. I've been assured that my cancer isn't a death sentence.

And, even if it was, I wouldn't know anything about it if I died.

But it would destroy Kirsty and the boys.

Shit, this is hard.

I'm worried about the treatment. The six weeks of combined radiotherapy and chemotherapy.

It's going to hurt.

A lot.

And I'm scared.

Quite honestly, I'm crapping myself.

I start my radiotherapy on 18th April – two weeks from now.

Talk about a countdown. This one will be a killer.

Pardon the pun.

How will I feel the night before it all begins?

I don't dare imagine. But, I'll be able to tell you all in just under a fortnight.

Watch this space.

I've got my third appointment for my tooth extraction. 7.30am this Thursday, 7th April. That could well knacker the rest of the day for writing.

I know what you're thinking. "So? Your health comes first."

No, my family comes first. I have to finish this book so that I don't risk losing the rest of the series.

Two weeks before my therapy starts. Then, maybe two weeks before it all kicks in and knocks me for six. That gives me about a month of writing time.

I have to make every day count.

Do other people with cancer have these worries?

Probably. I'm no-one special.

Stage four.

I wonder why it stops at four?

If my doctor had found this earlier, instead of thinking it was first mumps, and then a throat infection, what stage would I have been at?

How long have I had this thing?

I've had bad throats, chest infections and pneumonia for around four or five years now. Has that been this bastard all along?

The consultant said pneumonia can be caused by inhaling small fragments of food. This happens when you can't swallow properly and lapse into a coughing fit.

I've been doing that for at least the past four years.

For a while, whenever I ate, I ended up coughing. Sometimes to the point of blacking out. That's called cough syncope, and it happens when the heart suffers a lack of blood either on the way in or the way out - both meaning a lack of blood to the brain.

And bang - out you go.

I remember waking up to Kirsty thumping me on the back, shouting my name, presuming I was choking on my dinner. Arran was crying, and Sam was panicking, screaming "Dad! Dad! Oh, God! Dad!"

That was about four years ago.

Was that when this all started?

Have I had cancer for four years?

Does it really matter?

I'm here now.

And so is the cancer.

It's not even midnight yet, and I can already feel any hope

of tonight's sleep slipping away from me. My mind is racing, and I know it won't stop.

It very rarely does.

It's a genuine thing; a type of hyper-activity apparently. Where the brain doesn't shut down as it should at night.

It has a few bizarre side effects. The main one being is that I occasionally sleep with my eyes open. My Dad found me doing just that in my cot when I was just a baby. That was probably the first time.

It scared him!

I still do it from time to time. I know because I wake up with sore, red eyes.

I hope Kirsty doesn't catch me doing it. Not while all this is going on.

My depression is lurking again. I can feel it, like someone pulling a curtain inside my head. Making it dark inside.

I can't let it take over. Although it would be very easy right now just to crawl into bed and stay there, sleep or no sleep.

Just not get up again.

But, I can't do that. I have to stay positive.

I'm just not sure I know how.

NO PARKING

Today I received a clear sign that things are starting to get on top of me.

This morning, I had a planning meeting about my radiotherapy at Preston Hospital. If you read my recent posts, you may recall that details of this appointment were somehow sent to my parents old house, where I grew up.

Once we'd fixed the address mix-up with the unit on the telephone yesterday, they told me to come in today and park in Car Park 'L', right outside the cancer centre.

So, after dropping Sam at school, Kirsty and I drove to Preston, and found Car Park 'L'. But, there was a vast lorry sized scanning unit covering almost all of it. These travelling scanners and clinics are, of course, essential to many people - so I couldn't really complain.

Yet, for some reason, I found myself feeling quite staggeringly upset about not being able to park.

I figured I must just be nervous about the appointment.

So, I waited in the car while Kirsty nipped in to ask where we could park.

"You'll have to find somewhere else," was the reply. "But, whatever you do, don't park illegally, or you'll get a ticket."

Hmmm...

For the next hour, we drove around the hospital grounds, from car park to car park, looking for a space. They were all completely full, and most had cars queued up to enter just as soon as someone else left.

One in, one out.

Now, this was nothing more than a busy hospital having a limited amount of parking space for staff and visitors. Many, if not most, of the hospitals around the UK have similar problems. It's no biggie.

But I was really starting to get anxious.

And my mood didn't improve when we eventually found a spot, and I went to check in for my appointment. Once again, the receptionist had the wrong address. My old childhood address - a house I hadn't lived in for over 30 years. I corrected the mistake, again.

And, again, felt something bubble inside.

Then a thought occurred, and I spoke to the receptionist...

ME: "Why am I being treated in Preston?"

REC: "Because this is the nearest cancer centre to you."

ME: "Really?"

REC: "Yes, your address is just six miles away."

ME: "But, that's not my address, remember? I haven't lived there since I was 18 years old."

REC: "Oh, that's right."

ME: "I live 30 miles away now. It's a 60 mile round trip. Is there anywhere closer to me? Somewhere that might even have parking spaces?"

REC: "There's a cancer unit in Manchester, and they have a satellite unit in Oldham."

ME: "Oldham? You mean the Oldham that's about 13 miles from my house?"

REC: "Sorry?"

ME: "I have an Oldham postcode."

REC: "But..."

ME: "That's NOT my address!"

REC: "Oh, yes."

ME: "Can I be treated in Oldham instead?"

REC: "Is that what you want?"

ME: "Yes, please."

REC: "We'll arrange for an appointment to be sent out in the post."

ME: "To which address?"

REC: "What? Oh, hahaha!"

So, we left the unit and set off for home.

As we drove away from the hospital, Kirsty called my Macmillan nurse in Blackburn to explain what was now happening.

She was confused.

NURSE: "You can't be treated in Oldham. Oldham doesn't deal with head and neck cancers..."

ME: "What?"

NURSE: "They've never treated head and neck cancers. You shouldn't have been told you could go there."

Kirsty asked where I had to go for my treatment, in that case.

NURSE: "Preston."

KIRSTY: "But, we're just leaving Preston."

NURSE: "Then, you'll have to turn around. I'll call them and say you're on your way back."

At this point, I pulled over and took the phone. I explained about the parking situation at Preston Hospital and said that I didn't relish doing this five days a week, for six weeks.

NURSE: "How about if we arrange patient transport for you, then?"

ME: "OK, that would work. "Would they pick Kirsty and I up from home?"

NURSE: "Kirsty can't travel in patient transport, I'm afraid. You'd have to go by yourself."

And that was it.

Right then - everything hit home.

The last three months slammed right into me. The lump, the pain, the worry, the doctor's appointments, the blood tests, the biopsy, the scan, the diagnosis, the effect it's having on my kids, the loss of work, the lack of sleep, the impending treatment.

Everything.

All at once.

I'm slightly ashamed to say I completely broke down.

I thrust the phone back into Kirsty's hands and sobbed and sobbed and sobbed.

In my car, at the side of the road, in the middle of Preston.

It took Kirsty almost half an hour to calm me down.

I was a mess.

But, I had to pull myself together. I had to drive back to Preston Hospital, presumably abandon the car somewhere, and go back to the cancer unit for my now long overdue appointment.

UPDATE: The keen-eyed among you will notice that I have edited this post since first uploading it. That's because I didn't make myself clear in the original. The problem today was with me - not a single staff member at Preston Hospital.

I let the events of the past few weeks simmer just under the surface until such trivial issues as a lack of parking spaces and an address mix-up were enough to push me over the edge.

The staff at Preston hospital are wonderful, and they are not to be blamed in the slightest for my inability to cope with life's smallest of obstacles.

The cancer is starting to mess with my head.

Ha!

Geddit?

THE MASK

Today, I had a planning meeting with the radiotherapy team at the *Rosemere Cancer Centre* at Preston Hospital.

After a dodgy start to the day during which I got myself worked up over something as silly as the lack of available parking spaces (my emotions are still a little raw after the chaos of the past few weeks), I went in for my appointment.

The radiotherapy team couldn't have been friendlier, and they talked me through everything I needed to know in order to begin my treatment in two weeks' time.

This included being fitted for a mask.

The mask is used to hold your head and neck still while you are undergoing your treatment, and everyone has their own individual mask moulded.

They start out flat, then, after you've taken up your position on the table, the plastic mould is soaked in hot water, placed over your face and moulded into shape by a team of nurses.

You can possibly just make out that the mask is then pinned down to the table to keep you from moving at all.

I can't say it's the most comfortable thing I've ever worn (and I've been a panto dame many, many times), but it wasn't as terrifying as I'd imagined it would be.

Plus, the team were incredible.

I couldn't be in better hands.

The final task of the day was to give me a tattoo.

Yes, a tattoo!

This is so my body can be lined up in exactly the same position, session after session.

My first tattoo. Sitting proudly on my chest...

I feel like such a badass!

BIG BANG

The thing about battling an opponent like cancer is that, occasionally, the bad guy lands a punch or two.

And, sometimes, the villain forms a tag team with other nasties, just to make you feel worse than usual.

This happened yesterday when my stomach peg began to cause me problems. It was oozing pus and bleeding heavily. I took a picture for this blog but, believe me, you don't want to see it.

So, another trip to the doctor was required, where I discovered that the entry 'wound' was now infected. One thick dressing and a course of antibiotics later, and I was good to go.

Or so I thought.

This morning was the third attempt to remove one of my teeth prior to my treatment starting. Apparently, any tooth that looks as though it may be weak or unhealthy could cause major issues under the strain of radiotherapy - so they have to be pulled.

I had one such tooth - Upper 6 was its name. I'd had root

canal surgery performed on it back in the 1990s, but it didn't look as though it was strong enough to survive the attack of the x-rays.

I'd had two previous appointments to try to get this tooth out, but they'd both had to be postponed due to me being in too much pain. Today, I wasn't in too much pain.

Well, to begin with...

I turned up at the Day Surgery unit at Blackburn Hospital at 7.30am, as requested. From there, along with seven or so other men, we were taken to our ward and issued a bed.

I was asked to change into a gown - and to wear a pair of tight surgical stockings.

From there, I was taken into an operating theatre and laid on the operating table beneath the operating lights and beside operating machinery and trays of operating tools.

For a tooth.

Once I was hooked up to the machinery (the operating machinery, that is), the surgeons came in and explained that the tooth would be taken out under local anaesthetic.

Then, a mask was placed over my eyes.

I figured this was for one of two reasons...

- To protect my eyes from the bright lights of the operating theatre.
- To give the hospital staff the opportunity to sneak out and be replaced by the late, great Jeremy Beadle and his gang of wacky chums from 'Game for a Laugh'.

"We made you think you had cancer but instead, it's all a prank! Here's Henry Kelly to explain how we got the tumour into your throat in the first place..."

Sadly, it was to protect my eyes. *sigh*

And, so it all began...

Several rather painful injections later, my mouth and gums were numb, and the surgeons began to work. They explained that I would be able to feel quite a bit of pressure as they worked at the tooth - because, if there was one thing they didn't want to happen, it was-

BANG!

I actually jumped at the noise.

"What the hell was that?" I demanded, thinking that one of the operating lights had fallen from the operating ceiling.

But no, the sound had come from inside my own mouth.

It was my tooth.

It had shattered into dozens of pieces.

This was exactly what they didn't want to happen. Now, things were complicated. Really complicated.

"I'll need a blade, now," sighed one of the surgeons.

He sounded so disappointed that I almost apologised.

For the next thirty minutes, the surgeons cut into my gums and then pulled, broke, drilled and gouged the remaining slivers of tooth from its formerly happy home.

Ow!

Finally, it was done. The tooth was out.

Phew!

Then, one surgeon said to the other...

"Can you see that?"

"Yeah..."

Beneath the gauze, my eyes grew wide.

What was it? What they could see?

I asked, through my wooden, lifeless lips.

"Oh, we can see the end of your left sinus through the hole."

Good job I was lying down.

"We can stitch your gum across to cover it up but, what-ever you do, you mustn't blow your nose for the next two to three weeks."

Er, OK...

"If you blow your nose, it will increase the pressure on your sinus, and we'll have to operate again to relieve that."

I made a mental note to destroy anything resembling a tissue as soon as I got home.

An hour or so later, I was discharged - by which time, the anaesthetic was beginning to wear off.

OW!

Plus, all the pushing and shoving around in my mouth had agitated the cancery bits.

OW!

And the surgeons had inadvertently been resting their operating tools on my stomach during the procedure. Right on my infected stomach peg.

OW!

I'm back home now, and I'm going for a lie down.

I may get up again sometime in July...

SWEET TOOTH

I continue to receive good wishes via email, Facebook, Twitter and even through the post! I really am incredibly grateful.

Today's card came from *Coolabi*, the production company behind the *Scream Street* TV series. It included packs of official *Scream Street* sweets for Sam and Arran!

For those of you who may not know, I wrote a series of 13 books called *Scream Street*, featuring the adventures of a reluctant werewolf, a wannabe vampire and an action-hero mummy.

The books available all around the world, and are great fun to read - even if I do say so myself!

Why not buy one and find out for yourself? All royalties help!

Not long after the first books came out, I was approached by a TV company who wanted to turn them into a stop-motion television series. Five long years of planning, preparation and production later - and *Scream Street* premiered on CBBC (Children's BBC) here in the UK last October.

The animators - *Factory TM* - are making 52 episodes for

the first series alone. I've been along to watch the team in action - and the work they're doing is just fantastic!

I spent much of last year novelising some of the TV stories for publication. The two of those books - Uninvited Guests and Negatives Attract - were published yesterday in both the UK and the US!

I'm planning to keep writing for as long as the treatment allows; until it utterly wipes me out. I've got my dream job and nothing - not even cancer - is going to stop me from doing it.

UP, UP AND AWAY

U p again, unable to sleep because of the pain.

I've just taken some morphine (5ml, should you be interested), and that will kick in soon. It doesn't quite take the pain away, but numbs it enough for me to be able to function.

I had to sign the poisons book at the pharmacy when I picked up my prescription. A month ago, the strongest thing I'd take would be soluble paracetamol with codeine. Now I'm signing the poisons register and have a tattoo.

Cancer's turning me into a bad boy.

But, there are limits.

Several people have recommended marijuana as a way to ease the pain and even aid recovery - either in oil or its more regular form. But I won't do it.

I know it's not a powerful drug, and the stuff I'm prescribed for my high blood pressure is probably far more potent - but I've never taken any form of illegal drug in my life, and I don't want to start now.

Not because of its legality. I'm simply not interested. Never have been, never will. Just not my thing.

I can almost hear the critical among you ranting that I take a legal drug - in the form of alcohol - quite openly (or, at least, I did), and that's far worse than using marijuana can ever be.

That's probably the case. But - not interested.

I've heard many, many cases of people being rewarded with powerful pain relief through its use.

Wonderful. Still not interested.

I'm not being a snob, or a wimp, or a goody-goody, and I would never criticise anyone if they decided to use the stuff for medical or recreational purposes.

I'm just not interested.

My drink was whisky. Single malt. I gave up on beer several years ago as it just started to make me feel bloated and gassy.

Kirsty thinks I drank a lot, and she may be right. Sometimes I'd have three or four glasses in an evening with ice, which can equal half a bottle.

In the cold light of day, that is a lot. Certainly more than the government wants me to consume. All that units per week stuff.

Why am I worrying about this? Because it's possible - just possible - that drinking caused my cancer. I can never be certain that's the case, but then I can never be certain it isn't.

The doctors all asked if I smoke (no), have ever smoked (no). Then 'do you drink alcohol' was always the third question.

When I think of a 'heavy drinker', I think of some of the people I used to serve when I worked behind a pub bar many years ago. People who arrived straight from work, sat at the same position at the bar, every night, and downed one drink after another until it was closing time.

And, sometimes, they'd stay behind for a lock-in 'til two or three in the morning.

That wasn't me. I've never done that. But it doesn't stop me asking the question...

Did I do this to myself?

Am I directly responsible for my cancer?

As you'll know if you've read the other posts here, both my parents died from cancer. Other people in my close family have also had their own their own encounters with the disease.

That must count for something.

We're susceptible to it.

But the thought that I caused this myself - that I'm the reason for the stress and upset and worry my family are going through right now - is horrible.

If that's the case, then I deserve the agony of my forthcoming treatment.

Christ, that's a dark thought.

But then, it is the middle of the bloody night again - and you know what that does when you start thinking. What is it about the dark that makes your mind not only wander, but actively take the steps down to the unlit cellar?

Everyone else in the house is asleep. The vast majority of the country is in the same position. But, here and there - there are lights on in windows. People like me, unable to sleep because of pain or worry or plain old insomnia.

All of us having our worries amplified by the dark outside.

It's like a club. A club that none of us wanted to join.

I wonder what the t-shirt would look like?

I can feel the morphine kicking in now. Everything is turning dull. Fuzzy. There, but not sharp. Like background music or one of those apps you can get so you can listen to the rain to help you fall asleep.

I've got one of those. Kirsty and I use it quite frequently. It's really good. You can set it to rainfall, the sound of a babbling brook, forest noises - or even the ambience of a train station or coffee shop.

White noise, they call it.

White noise in the dark night.

I worry that these posts come across as self-pitying. Or, worse, playing on the emotions of you, dear reader.

I promise you that's not the case. I'm just trying to be honest about what I'm going through, and how it makes me feel.

My sister pointed out, quite correctly, that if my Mum had been around to read any of these blog entries, she'd have given me a good talking to. She'd have told me to pull myself up by my bootstraps. If I can't cope with the parking situation at a hospital, then how the hell will I get through six weeks of radiotherapy?

She's right, of course. Now's the time I have to be stronger than ever. Tougher than ever. Dwelling on 'what ifs', and 'how longs' won't do me any good at all.

I do try to be strong. Really. It's just that I'm scared.

Really scared.

I can't think of another time in my life that I've been so scared.

Oh, there have been moments. Watching first my Mum, then my Dad come closer and closer to passing away.

Passing away. I really couldn't bring myself to type the word 'dying' then. I even had to force myself in that last sentence.

There was also a time when Arran was much younger and we couldn't find him when we went to pick him up after school. We drove round and round, asked at reception, called his friends - but there was no sign of him. No-one knew where he was.

We found him - forty five minutes later - outside the playground of a different school nearby. There hadn't been any parking spaces outside his own school that day, so he'd kept on walking until he reached somewhere with a gap where we could pull in and collect him. He hadn't thought that we'd need to know where he was in order to do so.

Totally innocent, but the fear you go through when you can't find one of your kids...

That was scary.

But this... This is different. This is like a constant buzzing noise at the back of my head. And even if I manage to tune that out, every now and again...

WHAM!

It all comes back to me.

Hey Tommy - you've got cancer!

It's that word, isn't it?

That bastard word.

I'm a writer; I know how powerful words can be. But, that one...

It's a killer. In more ways than one.

DAD

Sitting up without sleep again (both sides of my mouth conspiring to keep me awake tonight), so I wanted to tell you about my Dad.

Brian Thomas Donbavand.

The best man I've ever known.

He worked incredibly hard to provide for his family. We were never rich. Quite the opposite, in fact. But, we never went hungry, and my brother, sister and I always got to go on school trips, etc.

My Dad was a coppersmith (think blacksmith, but with copper instead of iron or steel). He learned his trade in Liverpool, working as an apprentice with The Mersey Docks and Harbour Company where his dad (my Granddad) was a carpenter.

That wasn't his first choice of career. He wanted to join the police force but, back in the mid to late 1960s, his six-foot frame was turned away...

...because he wore glasses

That's the way it worked back then.

So, he joined thousands of other men - and some women - in tackling the dock road before and after work each day.

Years later, those same dock buildings would house clothes boutiques, swanky coffee shops and apartments people who grew up in Liverpool could never possibly afford.

My Dad lived at home with his parents - Thomas and Norah - and his brother and sister - Les and Shelagh - at 26 Captain's Lane in Bootle. That was a brilliant house. There was a brick shed and adjoining coal shed in the garden that had an old, thick tree growing behind it.

I spent a lot of my younger days climbing that tree in Nan and Granddad's back garden and surveying the world (well, Bootle) from that shed roof.

My Granddad had lost part of one of his thumbs thanks to a splinter of an unusual wood (I want to say Greenheart) and it had become infected. This shorter thumb always fascinated - and slightly scared - me as a kid.

In the course of things, my Dad met my Mum (then a nurse), they got married and along came yours truly. We lived with my Dad's parents in Captain's Lane to begin with but, from what I understand, it was a tense situation - so my Mum and Dad moved to a flat in Rutland Street.

My earliest memory is from there. I remember tables had been set up along the cobbled street, tables that were piled high with cakes and sandwiches. The event was the centennial or bicentennial of the local area, and I clearly recall sitting on my Mum's knee at the table, scoffing down a Bakewell tart, and chuckling with a girl in a pink dress as she ran around us.

My Mum told me that I would have been around 14 months old at the time.

After a few years, we moved first to the top flat in three storey block in Walsingham Close (where my sister, Sue, joined the family), and then to our first real home – 15 Haddon Avenue.

The house in Haddon Avenue was huge. Aside from the kitchen, it had three large rooms downstairs (which we rather imaginatively called The Front Room, The Middle Room and The Back Room) – at least until my Dad knocked the first two rooms through. This must have been sometime around my birthday, as I remember getting brick dust on my newly gifted football boots.

It was at this house that my brother, Bryan, completed the family. And it was also here that my Dad bought an old stand-up piano for the middle room (now the far end of the front room). It was old and battered, but it worked and I spent many happy hours banging dreadful tune after dreadful tune on it.

Other memories of Haddon Avenue: my sister filled butter tubs with water and mixed in petals from the flowers in the small garden (mainly snapdragons). This was her way of making 'perfume', which she used to add aroma to the beads from her childhood necklaces and bracelets.

I remember finding one of those beads on the floor on day. I wondered if it was one of the ones Sue had soaked in her home made perfume, so I raised my palm to my nose and sniffed hard.

We spent several hours at the local hospital before doctors could get that out.

This was also the house where – just as my Mum was getting us ready to go to school one morning – I opened a bag of spooky themed crisps known as Bones, and got one stuck in my throat. By the time we arrived at the hospital, this was being reported as 'he's got a bone stuck in his throat'.

Eventually, the crisp dissolved, and we went home.

I loved that house, and had a very happy childhood there. What I didn't know was that my Dad's workshop at the

Mersey Docks and Harbour Company was coming close to shutting down.

He had spent years there, working with copper piping to help make new boats and repair older ships. He'd occasionally take me down to the docks after he'd finished work, and point out which of the ships he'd worked on, telling me where in the world they were sailing off to with their precious cargo.

But that was about to come to an end.

My Dad needed a new job, which he found over 30 miles away at British Leyland, then still based in a town I'd never heard of - Leyland, in Lancashire.

So, we packed up and moved - from this big, weird house in Haddon Avenue, Liverpool to a smaller council house in Leyland.

25 Robin Hey.

This was where we lived next door to a murderer. Details later.

My Dad hated his job at British Leyland. There was just no imagination required. Where he'd had the chance to be creative in solving problems with his precious copper piping for Liverpool's great ships, here he sat at a machine all day and bent copper pipes into pre-designated shapes.

It drove him mad, and he lasted about six months before he moved to British Aerospace - first in Preston, and soon after at the Wharton Aerodrome.

From ships - to lorries - to fighter planes.

We moved house, too - to 7 Northlands, where my brother, sister and I would spend the remainder of our childhoods.

And where my Dad would continue with his practical jokes.

He convinced my then girlfriend that the M6 motorway was cobbled if you went further north than Preston.

One of his colleagues in the coppersmith's shop at

British Aerospace spent months going to night school to learn computer aided design so that he could better his prospects with the company. After the interview, this guy received a letter through the internal mail system explaining that he'd done well when meeting the interview panel, that they were impressed with his new qualifications and drive to learn....

Unfortunately, however, they weren't going to promote him to the design department because they didn't like his choice of tie.

Yep. Somehow, my Dad had persuaded one of the secretaries to type up the letter and sent it.

There was one guy who always borrowed my Dad's newspaper for his morning trip to the gents. So, my Dad planned ahead. One day, he bought TWO copies of the Daily Mirror, took one into work and kept the other inside a carrier bag on the top of the wardrobe for a year.

On the matching date the following year, he took the old newspaper into work and - as he always did - his mate nicked it and went off for a lengthy read.

He later said that he'd reached the what's on TV pages before he realised anything was wrong.

Years passed, we all grew older and, eventually, my brother, sister and I left home. My Dad retired and all seemed well, until we realised that my Mum was becoming increasingly unwell.

Despite my Dad growing older, his sense of humour remained the same. One time, back during the first Gulf War, I returned home from eight months away on the cruise ship where I worked. My Dad made me a cup of tea and handed over the post that had arrived since they'd last been down to Tilbury (where the ship docked in the UK) to see me.

My blood ran cold. There, in this pile of seemingly innocuous post, was a letter from the Ministry of Defence, postmarked from London. I opened it with trembling fingers, and my worst fears were realised.

Inside the envelope were my call-up papers to the army.

I was to be trained to join the ongoing fight in Kuwait.

The letter gave the time and date that I was to report to my training camp, and what I would need to bring along with me.

I'm fairly certain I was crying at this point. I'd only just embarked on a career at sea, and I was looking forward to many more years travelling the world and entertaining cruise ship passengers as I went.

Then the letter explained that, due to army cut backs, I would be required to buy my own tank. That wouldn't be a problem, however, as there was a superb range of 0% finance Chieftains currently available...

I nearly punched him!

My Dad was never meant to be alone. Losing my Mum hit him hard, and he struggled. Not with everyday life - he had us for that- but he struggled simply having to be by himself.

And then he met Barbara in an online chat forum. They quickly became good friends, and then more. They just clicked. Barbara made him very, very happy and - eventually, they moved into a house together in Southport.

He once told me that he'd been given a second chance.

Then came the news that he had prostate cancer.

It was a shock, but not unusual for a man of his age.

The treatment was complicated, and painful - but he battled through and was eventually given the all clear. We couldn't have been happier for him.

Life continued. He enjoyed his time at first Sue's wedding, then mine, and then Bryan's.

The family continued to grow - and my Dad loved every minute of it. As each new grandchild arrived, he seemed to be happier and happier. He and Barbara had a great social life, they enjoyed holidays abroad together and even opened a small DIY shop near their home in Southport.

I have a photo of my son, Sam (then around 6 or 7) is singing for his Granddad, and charging him a pound per song! I got my sense of humour from my Dad, and I guess it didn't stop there...

Then one day, around a year and half ago, he called me. I'd been to the cinema with Kirsty and the boys, and we'd just stepped outside into the sunlight when my 'phone rang.

DAD: "I've broken my arm, Tom."

ME: "What? How did you do that?"

He chuckled.

DAD: "By sneezing!"

It transpired that he'd been sitting down, had felt a sneeze coming, and was trying to get his handkerchief out of his pocket when the sneeze hit, sending a jolt through his body and breaking his arm.

It made for a good tale, and we all gently ribbed him about it for a while. Until it became clear that his arm wasn't healing.

He had x-rays and blood tests galore, but the bone simply wasn't knitting together. There was only one possible reason.

The cancer was back.

This time, it was in his bones. And it hit him hard. He was in excruciating pain, to the point where he could barely move around the house. Eventually, he was spending his entire day in a reclining chair in the living room.

I remember the first time I saw him in that chair. I'd been to visit him and Barbara many, many times. I'd seen him sit in that chair on several occasions. It was a normal, everyday chair.

But now, it looked as though the chair had grown too large for him. It swamped him on all sides and he looked so unbelievably small sitting in it.

That scared me a lot. Seeing my Dad looking so small.

By now, he wasn't eating much and he slept in the chair at night, rather than attempt the painful walk upstairs. It wasn't ideal, and everyone knew it.

So, my brother Bryan helped Barbara set up a bed in the living room for him.

For days, he resisted getting into it. Looking back, I think I now understand the reason why.

He knew he wouldn't get back out.

From then on, we all spent as much time as we could with him - sitting at his bedside, watching TV together and chatting. He started to sleep more and more, and so many of our visits with him were spent in silence, just holding his hand and listening to him breathe.

He died early in the morning of 15th June last year, 2015. We were all at his bedside with him.

Like my Mum, I miss him every single day, and I find myself thinking about him often. He was a wonderful man. Kind, caring, loving, strong.

Most of all, he was a family man.

He was my Dad.

MORE AND MORPHINE

I've had a LOT of pain around my stomach peg today, and that's what is keeping me awake tonight. I've just taken 5 ml of morphine, and I'm waiting for it to kick in.

The hole (for want of a better word) where the peg goes in is red raw again, and is starting to ooze with pus (sorry!) I finished my antibiotics today for an infection there, and I'm starting to wonder if I may need an extended course.

I can also feel a lump inside my stomach, just above the hole (access point? wound?) and that's where most of the pain is radiating from. I'm starting to worry that something is wrong - but that could just be the night time talking.

My tube was blocked earlier today. The sterile water I use to flush it just wasn't going in. So, we had to use the syringe to give it a bit of a boost, which did the trick.

Kirsty called the specialist peg nurse this afternoon and left messages, but we didn't get a reply. There's a 24 hour emergency number to call, which might be our next move.

Going to lie down again now and let the morphine do its work. I'll write an update later.

ALL IS CALM

The past few days have been very quiet. Aside from having to head back to my GP to have yet another infection in my stomach peg diagnosed and more antibiotics prescribed, very little has happened.

It's the calm before the storm.

My radiotherapy begins this coming Monday, 18th April. My appointment is at 4.15pm (although I'm hoping to switch my times to the mornings). The Wednesday of each week will be my chemo day.

I'm nervous, but just want to get started now.

Everyone continues to be incredibly kind and caring, with messages of support still coming in from friends, family – and many from complete strangers who have found the blog and enjoyed it.

I'm constantly amazed at just how many people have been through this horrible situation themselves, and how they've come away not only cancer free, but stronger in themselves.

Everyone has been fantastic.

My GP gave me her mobile 'phone number, and told me

to call whenever I needed to chat, or had a concern - even when she's away on holiday next week.

I received a lovely message from a couple I worked with on the *MV Kareliya* (one of the cruise liners I worked on in the early 90s). I haven't heard from them since I left the ship in 1993.

This afternoon I had a lovely visit from my Mum's sister, my wonderful Aunt Marie, who has always been there for me, especially since my Mum died. Her son, Mark, and his son, Josh, came with her. It was so wonderful to catch up with them.

Perhaps cancer has a positive side?

It unites people against a common enemy.

HOLD THE FRONT PAGE

Hello from the middle of the night again. Well, 5am to be precise - so we're well past the middle of the night.

Hello from the early hours of Sunday morning.

Without wanting to tempt fate - I think the antibiotics are working and the infection around my stomach tube is clearing up. However, as one area of pain eases, another blooms. Things are obviously getting worse inside my throat as my lower right gums are starting to swell and hurt.

The lump itself is practically pulsing with pain as I write this (maybe a touch over dramatic, but it's cool alliteration so I'll leave it in).

The big news is - I've made the news! The front page, to be precise. The front page of the *Rossendale Free Press*, no less.

I haven't taken a picture of the full story on page four, as I suspect it may be difficult to read on a screen, but here's how the story ran on the *Rossendale Free Press* website...

An award winning writer has launched a blog after being diagnosed with throat cancer.

Tommy Donbavand, 48, from Stacksteads, has already
received support from thousands of people around the world
as he battles illness.

The father-of-two currently writes *The Bash Street Kids* for
the *Beano* comic and is the creator of the CBBC animated
series *Scream Street*.

Tommy, who lives with wife Kirsty and sons Arran and
Sam, said he decided to write his blog to share details of his
diagnosis and upcoming treatment, and his fears and worries
about the future.

He said: "A few people suggested I start a blog so friends
and relatives could keep up with how I'm progressing.

"I thought the blog might be therapeutic for me, and
something I could hopefully look back at a year or two down
the line to remind me of what I've come through, so for it to
have resonated with so many people, who have taken the
time to contact me and send me well-wishes is incredibly
touching.

"It's both heart-warming and humbling to know that
people in the children's book industry are rallying around
behind me like this.

"My wife Kirsty has been wonderful in looking after me
despite her own poor health with Crohn's disease."

Tommy's friend Barry Hutchinson, who helped him set up
the site, said the response to his blog has been incredible.

He said: "Everyone knows someone who has been
affected by cancer, and Tommy has been able to put into
words what many sufferers may not be able to express
themselves."

After Tommy, who lives on Acre View, wrote about how
the illness and aggressive treatment plan have left his family
facing financial difficulties, the site's visitors were quick to

rally to his aid. So far more than 60 people – many complete strangers – have become 'patrons' of Tommy via Patreon.-com, sponsoring him on a monthly basis in return for exclusive written content.

Other top authors are also getting behind Tommy, who has written several official Dr Who comics and novels, with many offering to donate fees from their speaking events to help ease his money troubles during his gruelling treatment and recovery.

IT BEGINS...

I t's 5am on Monday 18th April - and I've barely slept yet again.

Only, this time, it hasn't been due to pain.

Later today, I have my first radiotherapy session at the Royal Preston Hospital. The first of 30 such sessions which, combined with what I've decided to call Chemo Wednesdays, will attempt to annihilate my cancer.

Which is nice.

However, this treatment is likely also to rob me - albeit temporarily - of the ability to talk, swallow or eat.

Which isn't quite so nice.

To say I'm nervous would be something of an understatement.

Don't get me wrong. I know I have to go through this in order to get well. It's just that I'm going to get a lot worse before that happens - and that's the part that's scaring me.

The doctors and nurses have warned that I will need speech therapy once my treatment is over. I'll also need to be taught how to swallow again.

They've said that I may emerge with different tastes, as

my taste buds are going to be completely burned away, and may not regrow the same.

I really hope I still like cheese!

I've also been warned that I may have a different voice when all this is over! This is down to the damage and self-repair my throat will have to endure.

A different voice! I can't get my head around that at all.

My neck is going to burn and blister - both on the inside and the outside. I won't be able to shave for six weeks or more, and I'll have to regularly apply cream to the affected area (albeit only on the outside).

I may have to start feeding through the tube - or peg - which has been fitted into my stomach. I have several boxes full of nutrient rich milkshakes ready and waiting to be poured directly into my stomach.

This one actually doesn't bother me as much. Since I had the peg fitted, I've had to flush it every day by pouring sterilised water down the tube (with Kirsty's help - it's practically impossible to do it by myself). This hasn't been as horrifying as I first thought it might be, and is actually becoming rather routine.

I wonder if the rest of the treatment will eventually feel just as ordinary?

The part I'm really not looking forward to is the destruction of my salivary glands. I won't be able to produce saliva at all and this, I've been told by many people, including several people who have undergone the same treatment, will result in my mouth and throat being coated with thick, stringy goo.

I physically shudder every time I think about it.

In a passing comment, one of my nurses mentioned the possibility of using artificial saliva! I can't think of a more disgusting product to try to force down my throat! I feel squeamish about it already.

So, I'm sitting up thinking and worrying - again.

Kirsty said that if that happens, I'm to wake her up and talk about it - but I can't do that to her. There's no point in two of us getting little to no sleep, especially when we've got the boys to look after.

Thankfully, they're still on their school holiday, so I get to have my first week of treatment sessions without having to worry about getting them to and from school and college.

5am. In 12 hours, the first session will be over. I will have been pinned to a table by my mask and bombarded with deadly x-rays for 15 minutes (yes, just 15 minutes - the one bit of good news in all this).

Then I have to do it all over again tomorrow, and the next day, and the next. For six long weeks.

Oh shit.

FIGHT NIGHT

Fight! Fight! Fight! Fight!

The battle has officially begun. Today at around 5.30pm, I had my first radiotherapy session. It wasn't the most fun 15 minutes I've ever had, but it wasn't horrific, either.

1 down, 29 to go.

I've started the fightback, cancer. You scared?

You damn well should be.

You're going down.

TWO DOWN

Not much to say today, I'm afraid. My radiotherapy session went smoothly enough.

2 down, 28 to go.

Or, R2/28

Although, there's a guy who comes along to get his treatment at about the same time as me. I saw him for the second time today.

He's a lookalike for my Dad!

I nearly jumped out my skin when I spotted him across the room yesterday. Today was easier, but still bizarre.

CRAZY CHEMO

I had to be at the cancer unit in Preston for 9am this morning, for my first of six chemotherapy sessions (every Wednesday).

C1/5, R3/27

I met my nurse for the day, who took Kirsty and I though what was going to happen, then I was shown to a large reclining chair at the far end of a ward. I got settled in, watched a DVD all about chemotherapy (really!), and then it was time to fit my cannula (the IV line to which my drip would be fitted).

And therein lay something of a problem. You see, I have a SEVERE lack of visible veins. Really, they're almost impossible to locate. Always have been. And whenever I've needed a cannula in the past (e.g. my frequent hospital stays for pneumonia over the past few years), fitting such a thing has always resulted in several false starts, calls for specialists from other wards and an arm like a pin-cushion.

However, my nurse wasn't going to be beaten so easily.

Several tourniquets and much hand shaking and slapping

later, a potential candidate was spotted and... BINGO! First time!

I want that nurse every Wednesday, please.

The first bag o' chemical magic fixed to my drip comprised of sterile water, packed with salts, antibiotics and no doubt many other wondrous marvels of the 21st century besides.

It was going in first to find and flush out any toxins I'd been selfishly hoarding in those hard to reach areas, such as the corners of my liver and kidneys, and would take a full two hours to take on board.

Followed by an hour of actual chemo stuff.

Followed by another two hours of the NHS's unique blend of 'flush out the crap' water.

To some people, the thought of sitting still for five hours straight would drive them insane. But to me it meant - uninterrupted, distraction-free writing!

I pulled my laptop from my bag, launched Scrivener and opened my work-in-progress. Cancer aside, I really couldn't have been happier at that moment in time.

Until, that is, my nurse reappeared at my side.

NURSE: "You going to watch a couple of movies on that?"

ME: "Actually no, I'm a writer and I thought I'd pass the time by getting some work done."

NURSE: "A writer?"

ME: "Yes!"

NURSE: "You mean, you'll be writing?

ME: "Yes!"

NURSE: "By typing?"

ME: "That is my preferred method of downloading stories from my brain to the page."

NURSE: "You can't type today. At least, not with your right hand."

ME: "My right hand?"

NURSE: "The hand where I fitted the cannula."

ME: "Oh. Why not?"

NURSE: "Have you ever had a cannula 'tissue' before?"

ME: "You mean when the line slips from the vein and pours the contents of the drip directly into your flesh instead? Yes, a few times. It really hurts."

NURSE: "Was that with antibiotics on the drip? For your pneumonia?"

ME: "Yep."

NURSE: "Chemo chemicals are a little different...

ME: "How?"

NURSE: "If you tissue while hooked up to today's drips - particularly the chemo drugs themselves - they will, first of all, burn a hole in the back of your hand and if not stopped, burn the flesh and skin all the way up to your shoulder."

ME: "Huh?!"

NURSE: "I've seen it happen; it's nasty. Really doesn't heal well."

ME: "Huh?!?!"

NURSE: "I'd keep your right hand as still as possible, if I were you."

So, I slowly closed the lid of my laptop, slid it back into my bag and reached for the solitaire app on my phone.

iPad, headphones and Netflix next week, methinks...

Once two hours had passed and I'd enjoyed the first of my two flushings of the day, it was time for the nurse to fetch and fit the drip filled with the nasty, cancer-bashing chemo chemicals.

WHICH CAME IN A BLACK BAG!

There may have been a skull and cross-bones printed on the side of the bag, but the bulky gloves of the nurse's fluorescent yellow hazmat suit make it difficult to see.

Besides, the lone church bell ringing far away in the distance was putting me off.

I jest, of course. Apart from the bit where it was...

GENUINELY IN A CHUFFING BLACK BAG!

I sat really still for the next hour.

Once the cursed pouch of acidic dragon's bile had been added to my bloodstream and was busy pumping its way through my heart and out to every corner of my body (what a jolly, jolly thought!), I had another two hours of cleansing to undergo.

By now, I was getting a little fidgety.

I'd tried to work by writing in my notebook with my left hand, but it looked like someone had scribbled their last will and testament while dangling off a sheer cliff face by their fingertips, the pen clenched between their teeth.

In Hebrew.

So, I just sat and waited for it all to be over with.

At one point things got so bad, I almost started a conversation with Kirsty.

I'M JOKING!

You can drop that expression! You know I don't mean it.

It would take more than five straight hours of mind-numbing boredom while my veins boiled with the addition of toxic chemicals for me to talk to Kirsty!

Ow!

Kirsty just read that bit over my shoulder as I wrote it and gave me a dead arm. 'Cos, you know, my body isn't suffering quite enough at the moment.

Ahem!

Eventually, it was all over. I was free to go home!

Except, I wasn't. Because now it was time for my radiotherapy session. I still had that to do!

Hahahaha!

This took longer than usual, too. My mask was somehow a little loose compared to yesterday, and Monday. The reason?

I've lost around half a stone since they first fitted it, and even dropped a couple of pounds this week alone.

The nurse told me to eat more.

I explained that, because of the pain in my mouth and throat, I was down to eating only soup.

She told me to add butter and melted cheese to my soup.

I said I'd think about it...

By the time the radiotherapy was over, I was exhausted. I found Kirsty in the waiting room, chatting to an elderly couple at the next table. She introduced me to them, and explained that the gentleman was here because he was suffering from the exact same cancer in exactly the same position as me.

I think it was the tiredness talking when I said the first thing that came into my mind...

"Congratulations!"

He didn't seem to find it as funny as I did.

Forget radiotherapy. Forget chemotherapy. I could feel that old geezer's eyes burning into the back of my head all the way to the car park.

If only we could have aimed his gaze directly at my cancer...

LOOKING UP

I t was my fourth radiotherapy session at the *Rosemere Cancer Foundation* in Preston today.

R4/26

I was feeling tired and run down following yesterday's inaugural chemotherapy treatment, but a visit from my amazingly good friend and former Buddy cast member and London flatmate, Alison, cheered me up to the point where I could finally drag myself off the couch and take on the world.

We had to go to Burnley Hospital first for Kirsty's latest appointment with her Crohn's specialist (we're such a healthy family!), then on to the wilds of Preston where, thanks to Kirsty being seen very quickly for a change, we arrived at 4pm for my 5.30pm appointment.

No problem. We grabbed a drink each, and settled down to read in the waiting room.

But, the eagle-eyed radiographers spotted that I had arrived far too early and hurried out to check that everything was OK. I explained that we were just running ahead of time for once, and thanked them for their concern. They said they would try to get in me in early, if they could.

I was seen at 5.35pm. Ah, well.

You may not know this but, as a lighting source in the room of big, scary machinery that fires plasma throwing stars at you (or something), there is a section of the ceiling that is made to look like the sky. You can just spot the tops of trees waving high above, and a few cotton wool wispy clouds floating across the clear blue sky.

Let me tell you, when you're lying on the thin bed-plank above, your face pinned to the end of it by a tightly-fitting meshed mask, looking up to see this albeit artificial sky can be very comforting.

That is, until you're raised higher and that three-pronged demon of technology starts rotating around your face, shrieking and buzzing and slowly obliterating the beauty of nature like a scene from your own personal Independence Day movie.

But, apart from that - it's great.

I had to have my mask re-seated twice today. Your head and neck have to be in EXACTLY the same position at every session in order for the treatment to work. This ain't no blunderbuss approach to burning out the badness within you, boy.

No, sir.

The team of three work to get me in the right spot, using fine-tuned laser-guided measuring equipment (really), and then they all bugger off to the safety of the next room while the 'you really don't want to be around when this shit kicks off' alarm sounds.

First, the machine revolves around you to take a three or four minute scan and check that you're millimetre perfect, position wise. If not, the trio of people to whom I will never be able to repay this debt hurry back in, unclip the mask and we start all over again.

There comes a point when, after the initial scan, that you lie there in silence, praying that it's all looking good on the bank of screens in the next room. If it is, the machinery kicks up again, twisting and turning and sounding like the Large Hadron Collider's attempt at an impression of a 1995 Packard Bell 56k baud rate modem.

That's your actual radiotherapy taking place right there.

If not, the radiographers come back in, and we try yet again.

It's a painstaking business and, no matter how frustrating it can feel for me, I try to remind myself that these wonderful people have been doing the same thing all day for patients just like me, trying hard to cure us of this terrible disease.

And, on only my fourth day, with a slightly different team on duty at each appointment so far, they still spotted that I had arrived early and came out to the waiting room to ask if I had any problems they could help me with.

How utterly amazing are people like that?

STATS TIME

So, that's the end of my first week of cancer treatment.
R5/25, C1/5

I really don't want to tempt fate, but I feel fine. Not as good as I did this morning, when I almost felt great. Then, today, the radiographers decided to target a new area of my cancer, so now I have some level of swelling and pain all over again.

Right now, I'd say I feel OK.

I've been checking out some of the statistics involved over the last few weeks, and they make quite interesting reading (who said this chapter wasn't sexy?) Check these babies out...

- Days since diagnosis: 36
- Days since diagnosis really sinking in: 22
- Days since diagnosis causing breakdown: 17
- Weight lost since diagnosis: 13 pounds
- Hours of sleep per night since diagnosis: 2 to 4
- Number of appointments since diagnosis: 19
- Number of days since treatment began: 5

- Miles driven to and from hospital this week alone: 300
- Parking fees paid at hospital this week alone: £22
- Number of posts written for this blog: 47
- Total number of blog visitors: 35,651
- Average number of daily visitors for blog posts when things are going well, and I'm reasonably chirpy: 400
- Average number of daily visitors for blog posts when I can't sleep, am depressed, or crying: 1,600
- Best example of this: Parking blog post, 5th April - 3,373 visitors
- Extra number of readers I'd get if I'd written this post while upset in the middle of the night: 2,000
- My level of gratitude for all the contact, support and help you amazing people have given me since this nightmare began: Impossible to measure!

Joking aside, I'm SO thankful for everyone who has taken the time to visit this blog, read my ramblings, comment on them, share them with online friends, and send me emails of support and advice.

It's almost impossible to believe that, as treatment has now started, the end could be in sight. The end of one of the scariest, world shattering, fast moving experiences of my entire life.

And thanks to you guys, I didn't have to face it alone.

You'll never know how much I appreciate that.

TAKE MY HEADACHE

OK, in an effort to keep this live and honest...

It's 5.19 am, and I've just woken up with a killer headache and some sort of goo bubbling out of my stomach peg hole. I've cleaned that up, and have some painkillers dissolving in a bottle of water next to me as I type.

I knew this feeling OK thing was too good to be true.

I didn't have soup for dinner tonight. I'm getting fed up with it. So, Kirsty made me some very mushy mashed potato and a couple of fish fingers. They were painful to eat, but I was determined to get through them.

After dinner I watched a bit of TV, then went to bed to read.

No, that's not entirely true...

After dinner I decided I wanted a glass of whisky.

Just a drop, over a couple of ice cubes - both to celebrate the end of my first week of treatment and the fact that I managed to finally finish my new book today.

But, there's a bit of problem I probably should have mentioned in my last post...

The stitches in my gum have finally melted, but they've left a hole. Remember when the hospital dental surgeons told me they could look through the spot where they had removed my tooth and see the end of my left sinus: Bang!

I was planning to tell the doctor about this at my first weekly review on Monday, just before my daily radiotherapy session. I know it will mean more gum stitches - which I'd rather not have, but hey ho.

As a result of this, whenever I've had a drink today, some of it has swished up that hole and dribbled out of my left nostril.

Which is not the end of the world, when it's water.

But ice cold whisky...

Holy Mary, Baby Jesus and all the little saints!!!

Kirsty found me hopping around the room, clutching at my face with a piece of kitchen towel and howling.

Please believe me, there are certain liquids that should not go through certain body parts in certain directions!

So, forget the whisky bit. I didn't really go anywhere (although the rest of the glass went down the sink).

Trying again...

After dinner I watched a bit of TV, then went to bed to read. I alternately read and dozed until the early hours when I got up to watch a video in my office to avoid disturbing Kirsty any longer. I'm not sure what time I staggered back to bed, half asleep - probably around 2-ish...

Until just now. I woke up with a jump, realised my stomach was wet, and then the pain made certain to intro-duce itself.

Bugger!

The tablets have dissolved now, so I'm going to take them (via a drinking straw so they go the right way around my head), and then go back to bed.

I really hope these past few days haven't led me into a false sense of security, and this is how I really should be feeling after my first week of treatment...

Sigh.

YOU AND WHOSE ARMY?

S omething incredible happened yesterday.

Something amazing.

I logged on to my computer at around 10.30am to notice a flurry of activity on Twitter around my name. Digging deeper, I found repeated references to two particular phrases: Tommy's Army, and the hashtag *#tommyVcancer*

These phrases spilled over to other social media outlets, such as Facebook - which was where I finally found out what was going on. It was all down to the brilliant Viv Dacosta - who has amassed a brave gathering of bloggers, book reviewers, authors and publishers to engage in a blog tour all about my books!

Viv and the crew worked tirelessly to keep the hashtag *#tommyVcancer* trending on Twitter for over five hours during the day! It was all I could but watch as visitor numbers grew on my blog, and more and more messages of support flooded in.

So, thank you Viv! Thank you everyone who took part in this, and who will take part in the forthcoming blog tour.

There haven't been many days recently when I've set at the computer and grinned - but yesterday was one of those days!

MEH!

I'll be honest with you - I spent much of today circling the drain. And that's despite yesterday's incredible show of support from book bloggers, readers, authors and just about everyone else connected to the publishing industry.

The promised fatigue has finally kicked in. I thought I was tired over the weekend, but trying to get up this morning was nigh-on impossible. The trouble was, I had to. I had to drive to Preston for today's radiotherapy session - R6/24 - followed by a progress meeting with my consultant.

The problem with fatigue is that... well, it isn't anything. It's not 'tired, so have a nap', and it's certainly not 'shattered after a period of hard work'.

It's just, as the youngsters of today say... MEH!

I don't like MEH!

I've never liked MEH!

Don't get me wrong - I love relaxing and chilling out and whiling away the hours as much as the next guy - but I want it to be my choice! Not because I don't have the energy to reach for my cup of tea.

And that's another thing! Everything has started tasting the same! And by the same, I mean the same as cardboard. Lord knows I'm restricted enough in what I can eat at the moment, but you'd think it might be possible to ascertain more than one flavour from a bowl of Scotch Broth, a Hazelnut Yoghurt and a cup of tea!

Nope.

All MEH!

And so it was when I met my consultant - Dr Biswas - for my progress meeting. He is great. Really great. He commented that he could see where the swelling in my face had started to reduce ("I've never seen you looking symmetrical before!"), chatted about how I'd coped with the first week's treatment and then admitted that he'd heard about my recent breakdown and had purposely hidden himself away from me all last week as a result!

He said that he knew he'd had to put me through so much, at such a tough pace, right after giving me some terrible news. He said he'd been expecting me to crack! And, when I did - he ordered the radiographers just to get me through the first week of treatment as swiftly as they could before he saw me again.

Then, he went on to tell me just how bad the next few weeks are going to be. No might be, or could be. It's going to be this way - and you're going to hate it. And, if I could give you a break, I would. But, I can't. Not if we want to get rid of this for a very long time.

I came out of that meeting grinning. I felt much better, despite the rotten prognosis. Because - once again - he'd been 100% honest with me. No bullshit whatsoever. I really, really like him.

So, week two is underway. I went to bed at 6.30pm this evening (yay, cancer!), and I've just got up to take my morphine before heading back for another attempt at sleep. I just thought I'd take the opportunity to check in while I was here.

KIRSTY

Another session of radiotherapy today.

R7/23

As ever, Kirsty was by my side to keep my spirits up, hold my hand when she saw I needed it, and generally teasing me to the point of giggles whenever I started to feel a bit down.

She's amazing.

Everyone who is diagnosed with cancer should be given a Kirsty.

Just not mine.

We met in the Black Bull pub in Bedlington, Northumberland - on karaoke night. Well, on a series of karaoke nights until I plucked up the courage to talk to her.

Eventually I asked for her number, and she told me that she didn't give it out.

I told her she couldn't possibly include me in that scenario...

I got the number and, 12 years later, here we are.

Very, very happy.

One thing you quickly notice about Kirsty is that she speaks her mind. Even if she doesn't always mean to.

She has... opinions.

About everything.

Nothing nasty, or cruel. She just says it as she sees it. Which doesn't always go down well. But, that's just who she is.

I wouldn't have her any other way.

When she was pregnant with Sam, I used to wonder if it was him I could feel moving around inside her. Or if it was simply the next batch of opinions, lining themselves up to be set free!

I won't go into too many details here, but she's not had an easy life. As a child, she was often mistreated and frequently hurt and abused.

She once asked a social worker how she could be certain she would never treat her own children in the same way. The social worker said the mere fact she was asking that question meant she never would.

She's an amazing Mum to both Arran and Sam.

Not many people know this, but she has two other children, as well. Two daughters who - sadly - have been so poisoned against her by other family members, that she hasn't seen them or spoken to them in many years.

It hurts her every single day.

Yet, she somehow continues to be this beautiful, uplifting person.

Again, few details, but...

When she was a child, Kirsty and her younger brother were put into a children's home for a while. She says it was one of the happiest periods of her life.

During their stay, a visiting family wanted to adopt Kirsty's brother - but not her. Splitting up siblings wasn't necessarily seen as a bad thing in those days.

So her brother (who I'll call 'G') was adopted, and she lost touch with him. Until one day, around eight years ago, when he contacted her out of the blue via Facebook.

Can you imagine how happy she was?

G now had a family of his own. He and Kirsty spent several happy weeks swapping stories and photographs. Until we discovered a terrible secret.

This was a fake account.

It wasn't G at all.

It was another member of her family, pretending to be him.

That's the sort of thing she's had to deal with.

That's how strong she's had to be.

And now she's there for me.

I love her. She's mine. Get your own.

IT'S MURDER

M y second day of chemotherapy today, followed by another radiotherapy session...
         C2/4, R8,22
We arrived at the cancer unit in Preston to find ourselves sitting next to a couple of Bamber Bridge - just a few miles away. We soon began to chat (no-one stays shy when you all have something as large and bastard-shaped as cancer in common), and I happened to mention that I had grown up in a particular area of Leyland.

"Ah!" said the guy. "The handless corpse!"

The Handless Corpse was the name the national TV and press gave to the murder case I alluded to in an earlier post.

I said I would come back to it and explain more, so here we go...

When we first moved from Liverpool to Leyland in 1979, we lived on an estate just off Slater Lane called Robin Hey. We moved into number 25. It was a smaller house than we'd been used to, but still plenty of room for the five of us, and my sister, brother and I had a big garden to play in.

Our next door neighbours were a young couple ‑ Andy

and Barbara, and their new-born baby. They were pleasant people. Andy made model aircraft and liked showing them off to me and my sister, and we occasionally played games of badminton over the garden fence with him.

They had a lot of visitors who, if Andy and Barbara weren't in, would frequently wait in our house until they were home; my Mum would make them cups of tea and chat (she was very good at chatting!)

One such visitor was a guy called Marty from New Zealand. I remember he was dressed in a white suit the first time I met him at our kitchen table. Strange the things that stick in your mind.

Months passed without any kind of event until early one morning - just before 7am - a dozen or so cars screeched into the cul-de-sac side road where our house was located.

Men jumped out of the cars, spotted the number 24 on the nearest house and raced up our front path, presuming the houses would be numbered as odds and evens, and that we were number 26.

But, the houses were numbered sequentially on Robin Hey - we were at number 25, and 26 was next door where Andy and Barbara lived.

My Dad was in the middle of brushing his teeth when a gang of armed police hammered on the front door. He said he almost swallowed his toothbrush.

The mistake soon realised, everyone charged to the next house along, the door was kicked in - and we soon found ourselves living right on top of to an active crime scene.

Of course at the time, we had no idea what was going on - but it wasn't long before the press began to arrive en-masse, and we were able to find out.

There had been a newspaper story the week before in which two recreational scuba divers had been exploring a nearby flooded quarry - Ecclestone Delph. The place was full of junk - old fridges, abandoned cars, etc. So, it was a popular location for local divers.

However, on this occasion, the shocked scuba enthusiasts had discovered more than they bargained for beneath the surface.

They found a body, caught on a ledge just a few metres down. If it had missed and sunk lower, it may never have been found.

Obviously, the police gave little away, but the story was to progress over the following few days to explain that the victim's teeth had been destroyed, and both his hands had been cut off and remained missing - both deformations a way of obscuring the identity of the individual.

In an attempt at gathering names, the man's face was rebuilt and posters of this death mask were printed to pass around in pubs and clubs. The search for the missing hands - and vital fingerprints (this was well before modern DNA testing), went onto overdrive.

The press called the case, *The Handless Corpse*.

They postulated the murder was a professional hit, ordered from the top ranks of an international drug ring.

But that wasn't exactly the case.

Thanks to a unique medallion the victim was wearing, he was soon identified as Martin Johnstone - a New Zealand drug dealer who had, apparently, been a little too flashy with his earnings and whose behaviour had overstepped the mark.

The guy in white suit I'd met in my kitchen.

He'd been murdered by Andy. My next door neighbour.

How do I know? Because Barbara and her friend, Julie, walked into the police station in Leyland a few days later and confessed.

Andy had run when he realised that he was about to given up. For the next week or two, police staged a scene at number

26 Robin Hey. A lookalike female police officer moved in, along with several armed - and hidden - personnel. They were there to trick Andy in case he came back to the house.

Parked in the streets outside were cars full of detectives and plain-clothed officers. My mum used to send me over with flasks of tea and sandwiches for them. One of the officers threatened to arrest me if I didn't take the 50p tip he offered me!

Andy was caught re-entering the UK at Heathrow Airport some time later, tried and convicted. He was given life in prison.

Postscript one...

In 1992, a TV movie was made about the story called All Good Friends. Much of the footage was shot in and around the original houses and the quarry where the body was dumped.

I watched the film when it was released on DVD.

At one point, shortly after the murder, Victor McGuire as Andy is at home, mulling over what he has done when there is a sudden noise, causing him to panic.

"Relax!" says another character. "It's just the kids next door..."

i.e. me, my sister and brother!

Postscript two...

It has often been said that Andy had no choice in killing Marty. That he would have been targeted if he had not gone through with his orders. I don't know if that is true or not.

From what I believe, Andy left prison a broken man, and was taken in by his elderly parents who continue to care for him.

As an author - and someone who was there when all this was happening, I've occasionally wondered whether I should write the book that tells the story from Andy's perspective.

Postscript three...

I'll begin this final section by saying that I have absolutely no belief in the work of mediums, astrologers, fortune tellers or anyone else who professes to be able to talk to the dead or see the future - for profit or otherwise. I think they are scandalous, wicked people, out to prey on the weak and unhappy.

That said...

The year is now 2005. I've just met Kirsty and we've been on a couple of dates. On this particular night, there was a 'spiritualist' performing above a pub in Bedlington, where we both lived. Kirsty wanted to go along but I wasn't so keen, for the reasons stated above.

However, I liked her and didn't want the night to end early, so I went with her.

The first 20 minutes were laughable, to the point where I even suspected the guy might be a parody act.

"Does anyone know a John? John? Could be Jack? John or Jack? How about Jerry? It begins with J. It sounds like a J, at least. It could be a K. Keith? Does anyone know a Keith? Kenneth? What about a Steven...?"

It was going to be a long night.

Then, around 20 minutes in, the guy pauses and points to the row at the back where Kirsty and I are sitting...

MEDIUM: "Someone there is a writer."

I nearly shat myself.

ME: "Er... yes."

MEDIUM: "And you're considering a new book..."

ME: "Yes."

MEDIUM: "About some very bad people."

ME: (Croak) "Yes."

MEDIUM: "He's telling you to leave it alone."

ME: "He?"

MEDIUM: "He says these people are too dangerous. That they'll get what they deserve in the due course of time. He's telling you to go no further."

ME: "---"

Then, as quickly as it had happened, he was back to the front row. "Does anyone here ever have an Auntie Carol? Caroline? Claire? Does anyone here know a woman of any description?"

I didn't take a breath until I was at the bar.

In a pub two streets away.

And I've just scared myself writing about it again now.

Maybe I'd be better off sticking to books about reluctant werewolves and action hero mummies?!

HEAR THE ECHO

Another day, another radiotherapy session down.
R9/21
I met a woman at the centre today who was there for her final RT session after fifteen solid weeks of treatment. Fifteen weeks! The chemo sessions made her so ill, they had to scrap them and just blast her cancer with x-rays.

Yikes!

Something I've come to learn over the past six weeks since I was first diagnosed (yep, this madness only started six weeks ago!) is that everyone's story is unique. There isn't really one such thing as 'cancer', and there certainly isn't one person's journey through treatment.

I received a lovely email from the chairman of a Head and Neck Cancer Support Group in Devon today. I really hadn't realised such things existed, but I can see how helpful they might be. Plymouth may be a bit of a stretch for visits however, so I'll ask for details of local groups at my session tomorrow.

I got my parking permit, too!

Also, I made the *Liverpool Echo*. Here's what they had to say...

Liverpool creator of CBBC's *Scream Street* gets worldwide support after starting cancer blog

BY DAWN COLLINSON

The Liverpool creator of hit CBBC animated series *Scream Street* has had support from around the world after starting a blog detailing his battle against cancer.

Tommy Donbavand from Orrell Park is an award-winning author and writer of *The Bash Street Kids* for *The Beano* comic.

But most recently he's been penning *Tommy V Cancer*, giving an honest personal account of the ups and downs of his diagnosis and treatment.

The 48-year-old dad of two was diagnosed with inoperable throat cancer in March this year and is currently in the middle of six weeks of intensive radiotherapy and chemotherapy which, he's been warned, may leave him unable to talk or eat and suffering extreme pain for months.

He explains: "In order to allow me to understand my illness better, and to help people who may find themselves in a similar situation, I started a blog to chart my battle against this horrific disease.

"A few people suggested it so friends and relatives could keep up with how I'm progressing."

Initially he thought the *Tommy V Cancer* blog would go no further than them, as well as answering questions his sons, 16-year-old Arran and Sam, 9, might be worried about asking directly.

But Tommy, who has written several official *Doctor Who* comics and novels, been amazed to receive support from thousands of people around the world, including fans and fellow best-selling writers.

They have been following his updates, posting comments, and sending him emails urging him to keep fighting back.

"The response has been incredible," says Tommy's friend, Barry Hutchison, who helped set up the site. "Everyone knows someone who has been affected by cancer, and Tommy has been able to put into words what many sufferers may not be able to express themselves."

Not only have they offered words of encouragement, they rallied to his help financially too when he revealed that the illness and aggressive treatment plan have left his family facing financial difficulties.

So far more than 60 people – many complete strangers – have become patrons of Tommy via *Patreon.com*, sponsoring him on a monthly basis in return for exclusive written content.

Other top authors are also getting behind him, with many offering to donate fees from their speaking events to help ease his money worries during months of gruelling treatment and recovery.

"I thought the blog might be therapeutic for me, and something I could hopefully look back at a year or two down the line to remind me of what I've come through," says Tommy. "So for it to have resonated with so many people, who've taken the time to contact me and send me well-wishes, is incredibly touching."

Now, I'm off to order a bottle of artificial saliva. What do you reckon? Lemon, or Mint?

ARRAN

So, that's week two of my chemotherapy and radiotherapy treatment over!

R10/20, C2/4

I almost didn't make it to the hospital today. We woke up to find out that it had been snowing all night and - as the Rossendale Valley is twinned with Narnia - we were snowed in.

Kirsty called the hospital to ask what the procedure was. The radiography department insisted that I make it in, switching my appointment from this morning to this afternoon and - if required - this evening.

Under no circumstances was I to miss this session.

Thankfully, the snow thawed enough for me to be able to get the car off the drive in the early afternoon, so I was at my radiotherapy session for around 3pm.

I'll write more about that later...

I want to cover a different topic in this post because today is quite a special day in the Donbavand household. It's my older son, Arran's, birthday. He's 17!

I'm very proud of Arran for many reasons, among the main of which is this little secret...

I'm not Arran's real Dad.

Well, not in the biological sense, at any rate. That spectacular waste of DNA didn't stick around to get to know him.

I first met Arran when I met his Mum, Kirsty. He was 6 years old. And he had a lot of problems.

The main issue was that, like his two older sisters, he was separated from his Mum - although that wasn't anything to do with her.

If you've been following my posts, you'll have come to realise that Kirsty's immediate family were... well, let's just say they never had her interests at heart.

In fact, I'd go so far as to say they actively disliked her.

And that's putting it mildly.

She was abused at home, spent time in a children's home while her Mum was in prison, then separated from her brother when he was adopted away. For more on that, see: Kirsty

By the time I met Kirsty, she had three children - all of whom lived in Coventry with her Mum.

As I now know is common in cases of domestic abuse, Kirsty switched between moving out, starting to get a new life - then returning to the abusive environment whenever she was pressured to do so.

It was like a bad marriage, only with her own mother.

When I showed up, Kirsty was living alone in Bedlington, Northumberland.

Why? Because at the end of yet another cycle of abuse, she had left to find yet another place to stay - only to return to collect her kids and discover that her family had been to court, claimed she had abandoned them, and received a residency order to keep them away from her.

She was allowed to travel to Coventry to visit her own children once or twice a month - and that was if and when the family were bothered to bring them along to the contact sessions.

As you can imagine, this was tearing her apart.

But if things were bad for Kirsty, they were a lot worse for Arran. You see, his older sisters were savvy enough to realise that if they played along with the family's anti-Kirsty tirade, they got an easy life.

Arran, however, just wanted to be with his Mum. And they treated him horribly for it.

Many was the time we'd collect him for a weekend contact and he'd tell us he'd been hit, or that he didn't have his glasses because they'd been slapped off his face and broken. Allegations which, of course, were all strenuously denied in court.

But, there was no way that Kirsty and I were going to let him down. We fought on in court for another three years to have his residency changed.

It was a horrible period of time. As if going to court regularly wasn't bad enough, Kirsty's family started to turn on me for supporting her.

I received a solicitor's letter claiming I had physically assaulted Kirsty's Mum in the court waiting room.

Questions were raised before the judge as to whether it was safe to leave me alone with children.

And my parents, siblings and even publishers received 'anonymous' emails claiming that I was being investigated by police for soliciting prostitutes.

Horrible. But we weren't going to give up on Arran.

Eventually, we won. He was nine years old when he finally came to live with us, only a few weeks after Sam was born.

Suddenly, I had a family!

And the best part of it was, because Arran looked a little bit like me, no-one ever suspected that I wasn't his real

Dad. In fact, it's something we don't even think about these days.

However, despite the happiness, it was the that I began to realise the true scope of Arran's problems.

He suffers from DCD (a developmental co-ordination disorder which used to be known as Dyspraxia - think all over dyslexia), he has hyper-flexive joints, bad asthma, and he's almost blind in one eye.

We were also told that, due to his limited abilities, he would very likely never be able to travel by himself. He was at risk of getting lost, taking the wrong bus, or even getting into a stranger's car. I would have to drive him everywhere.

Because his 'guardians' hadn't been interested in raising him - only using him as a tool through which to hurt Kirsty - he still couldn't read or write, and his speech was so poor that more often than not, I couldn't understand what he was saying.

They had never helped with homework, and so he was years behind at his new school just around the corner from us.

Yet, he remained so upbeat, and happy to back with his Mum.

So, I sat him down and made him a promise. I promised that, if we worked hard together, I would teach him to read and write, and we'd work hard on his speech. The plan was that, by the time he reached secondary school at 11, no-one would ever know he'd had these problems.

And he did it. Not me, not we. He did it.

By the time we moved to Lancashire, he joined his new primary school in year 5 able to read, write, talk - and he was only a little distance behind his year group.

We had spent every day playing word games, reading together, practising tongue twisters, spelling lists, writing stories and much, much more.

Please note, I'm not including these examples to ridicule Arran in any way - it's just a fun way to show his progress. He laughs about them just as much as we do. Honest!

Thanks to his DCD, Arran used to have a very poor memory (we invented memory games to help with that!), and quite often he would grasp somewhere around 10% of a subject, forget the rest and fill in the blanks himself.

This led to some very interesting after school comments...

ARRAN: "Jesus was born in a gingerbread house in space, Dad!"

ME: "Hmm... I'm pretty sure, he wasn't."

ARRAN: "Yeah - Miss told us!"

This transpired to be the fact that there is a star painted on the ground where the stable is supposed to have stood in Bethlehem. A house on a star, therefore in space. I've still no idea where the gingerbread bit came from.

ARRAN: "We're writing about the story of Easter, Dad!"

ME: "Are you?"

ARRAN: "Yeah, it's really horrible!"

ME: "True, it does come with its very own gory ending..."

ARRAN: "Too right! Jesus was *juicified*!"

And, my all-time favourite...

He was 100% correct in his written homework about Charles Dickens's classic, A Christmas Carol. He just had trouble spelling the word 'visited'...

ARRAN: "Scrooge was fisted by three ghosts during the night."

I'll just leave that image there for you... ;)

Secondary school was where Arran was really challenged. He was initially missed off the special educational needs list due to an error, and things didn't go much better from there.

He battled through year 7, keeping up with his school-work and doing well. Then, early in year 8, his asthma took a serious turn for the worse, and he missed a few weeks from school.

Kirsty was telephoned almost constantly by his head of year and, despite being able to hear Arran's horrific hacking cough in the background and the fact that we had a note from the doctor, she insisted we bring him to school the very next day.

"He's not well enough!" Kirsty insisted.

"I understand that," came the reply, "but if he comes in and tries, then I can find him, see he's not well and send him home. That at least gets him a mark in the register."

So, against our better judgement, we drove Arran to school the next day. He struggled through his first few lessons (despite teachers complaining about the volume of his coughing!), then made his way to see the head of year first thing after lunch.

We'd told him how this would go; she would call us to collect him, and he'd get his mark in the register.

But that didn't happen.

His head of year took one look at him, said "I'll decide if you're ill or not!", and sent him straight back to class.

He was in tears and still wheezing when we finally picked him up at the end of the school day.

I demanded a meeting with the head of year. She agreed, on the promise of prosecuting Kirsty and I for keeping Arran at home for an extended period of time.

I was ready for this.

My first question was to ask the head of year for a list of her medical qualifications. She blinked in surprise, then assured me that as a teacher, she didn't need medical qualifications.

"So, how can you possibly tell Arran that you will decide whether he is ill or not?"

Shields were raised at that point...

I asked her what she knew of Arran's special educational needs and health problems.

"Only what's on the school files," she said.

"Show me what that says," I continued.

With a sneer, she logged into the school computer system, and brought up Arran's file...

...which was completely empty.

They'd lost everything.

There was no mention of his DCD, dyspraxia, joint problems, eyesight issues, chronic asthma. Nothing.

Just a blank screen.

You've never seen anybody back-pedal as quickly as that woman!

It was fantastic!

By the time we left the school, Arran had been called out of class for an apology, and he was shown around a section called Stage Two. Normally reserved for disruptive pupils, Arran was offered a separate desk away from the rowdy kids in there along with a permanent pass for him to simply get up, leave class and work alone if he ever felt unwell.

He was also given a laptop for his schoolwork, and extra time was added to all his exams from that day forward.

Chalk one-up for the Donbavands!

Arran continued to work hard, and get exemplary reports throughout his time at that school. He had decided that he wanted to work in the computer games industry, and chose his options based on that career.

His next move, after taking his GCSEs, would be to move up into sixth form and do A Levels in Physics and Mathematics.

A place was set aside for him.

Physics and Maths A Levels - for the kid who couldn't read or write just seven years earlier. He had to work SO hard to get there, harder than any of his classmates who didn't have the problems he faced every single day.

He passed all his GCSEs. Seven Cs, and two Bs.

We were so proud of him.

Then came the day he went in to take up his sixth form place. I drove us up to the school but, because it was so busy, there was no room to park. So, Kirsty took him in to sign up, and I drove around the block, returning to collect them a short while later.

To find Arran in tears.

The head of sixth form had told Kirsty - in front of our son - that he didn't believe Arran had an aptitude for learning, and they were rescinding his previously offered position in the sixth form.

Never has an individual been so lucky that I had nowhere to park my car!

But, we weren't beaten. We raced home and immediately went online, discovering that Accrington College - a mere ten miles away - was running a course in computer games design and programming.

And today was the open day.

We took Arran in for an interview where they were so impressed with him - and his exam results - that they skipped him passed the entire first year of the course, and put him straight into the second level.

Many of the students were also having to retake certain GCSEs alongside their new course - but not Arran. His English and Maths results were just fine.

Now, two full terms later, Arran leaves the house at 7am to head to college on the bus every day. On his own. He hasn't got lost once.

His tutors tell us he's expected to ace his course with at least four distinctions. From there, he plans to switch to the college's own software development course before either university, or a job in the games industry.

Arran hasn't really spoken to me about my cancer since I was diagnosed. He's sat and listened whenever I've news to share with the family and he helps look after 9yo Sam when I have my hospital appointments (the two of them are as thick as thieves, most of the time) - but that's about it.

I suspect he's hoping that, if he doesn't talk about it, it isn't really there. Well, it is really there, mate. So, if you read this - a) clear the empty drinks cans out of your room, b) - get your hair cut, and c) - come and talk to me any time at all.

Well, that's my son. That's my Arran. That's how hard he was worked to get to where and who is today - a wonderful, kind, intelligent young man with a dazzling future ahead of him.

He's my hero.

BRAVE HEART

I've received many, many messages of support since my battle against cancer began - and they have all been special. Some of them are from family, others from friends, and so many from complete strangers who have taken time out of their day to wish me their best and offer their thoughts and prayers.

This message, however, is something special - and I have the wonderful Paul Magrs to thanks for it. As you probably know, I'm a huge fan of *Doctor Who*, so when this arrived on my Facebook page, I was incredibly excited...

"Dear Tommy,

So sorry to hear your bad news, but the very best of luck with it. As a great man once said: brave heart!

Much love,

Russell T Davies"

For those of you who may not know, RTD is the writer/showrunner who brought the series back to TV after just over 15 years in the wilderness, barring the very well-meaning, but flawed, TV movie (which, however, did bring us the legend that is Paul McGann as the Eighth Doctor).

On 6th December 1989, the Seventh Doctor and Ace strolled away from the camera at the end of the third and final episode of *Survival*, on to further unseen adventures. Then, on 26th March 2005, the Ninth Doctor met Rose in, er... *Rose*, and the fun continued.

Unfortunately, some people criticised Russell for his writing on the series, but I thought his scripts were incredible, and his sheer love for the concept and its main character shone through in every single story. He worked incredibly hard to resurrect my favourite TV show and, for that, I'll be forever grateful.

I'm now even more grateful, thanks to the message above.

ON THE SIDE

Holy crap in a bucket!

The long-promised side effects from the radiotherapy have all shown up on the doorstep at once, and they've brought a few friends along for the stay.

In case you're about to begin radiotherapy for head and neck cancer, you may want to skip this post. I don't want to scare you, but I promised I would be open and honest with every single entry, and today's truths are - heh - a little hard to swallow.

- I can almost no longer swallow. My throat appears to have been filled with a mixture of razor blades and those dagger things Raphael carries in episodes of Teenage Mutant Ninja Turtles. Sai. They're called Sai. A river of pain runs from the back of my nose, down into the dark, drool-free depths.
- My mouth is filled with ulcers. I tried count them at one point in the night but a), I couldn't open my lips wide enough to see them all in the mirror and

b), I almost dozed off half-way through in some bizarre sheep jumping over the gate/blister-strewn waking nightmare.

- My tongue is so swollen, I can barely speak. It feels like I have one of those large Italian sausages wedged down my mouth and throat. You know the kind - them ones you see hanging up behind the counter in the butcher's shop, but never seem to be sold, and you sometimes think about buying one just to try it, but then you realise you have no idea what on earth they're really called so how could you ask for it, and what if they're made of plastic and just for display and that would make you look like a fool, so you just buy four slices of corned beef instead and go home for a bit of a cry. Or, is that just me? (If anyone reading this is now smirking at the words 'large Italian sausages', don't let the door hit you on the way out. We don't need your kind in here, thank you.)

- My taste-buds have been fried. ALL taste is now gone, except for my innate fashion sense, which is clinging on by a few, weak tendons.

- Salivary glands - utterly burned away and missing in action. My mouth is as dry as a nun's laundry basket. I have a prescription for artificial saliva to collect from the chemist today, which I will have to pick up in dark glasses and some form of disguise.

- Seriously! Artificial saliva?! I once ate dog when I was in a restaurant in Brazil. Actual dog! To be fair, it wasn't until the word 'Labrador' was printed on the receipt that I knew I'd eaten dog, and yet the thought of this stuff turns my stomach into much angrier shapes.

Large Italian Sausages. Heh-heh!
And here are a couple of the bonus prizes...

- Chronic constipation. I don't have many pleasures left in life at the moment. Gone is the warm kiss of a wee dram as it twinkles a golden path down my throat. Lost is the taste of a good medium-rare steak, smothered in pungent blue cheese sauce. Forgotten is the ability to fling open the windows and tell the kids in the street where to go for hitting my car with their bastard football yet again. Cancer - please let me keep the gentle thrill of playing solitaire on my phone while I have a nice poo!

- My stomach peg is infected - AGAIN! Hahaha! You couldn't make this stuff up. What's more, the nurse is coming out to 'reseat and rotate' it on Tuesday. You see, if you have a stomach peg in for too long, the lining of your stomach accepts the inner workings as a new part of your body and grows over it. The scientific way to stop this from happening is to give a good old tug on the bugger, tear it free and let nature start all over again. You cannot imagine how much I'm looking forward to that.

- Poor eyesight. What? How?! I mean, where did that one spring from? How can having cancer in my throat affect my eyesight? Actually, don't answer that - I don't want to know. It would probably end up me having to have an artificial eyeball fitted so I could pour milkshake nutrients directly into my brain, or something.

- I can't blow raspberries. I was chatting to my two year old niece, Eliza, on FaceTime last night (well, croaking to her), and I thought the least I could do to make her laugh as the 'funny uncle' was to fire a good old raspberry out. Nothing. Silence. I spat what precious little saliva I had left all over my computer keyboard.

- Heartbeat. I can feel every thump of my heart pulsing in my throat. To be fair, this is a side-effect I'd like to hide rather than get rid of completely.

So, that's me today. I suspected things were about to take a turn for the worse as yesterday's RT session was the first I'd come out of in pain. Not through the Invisible Lasers of Dimension X themselves, but just from the way my mask has started to press down in different areas of my head and throat.

Still - it could be worse, couldn't it? I could have received the notes back from my editor on the first draft of my new book which I struggled to complete and send in last week, and the notes could be so heavy and demanding that my inbox actually cried out in pain for a few seconds when the email arrived, and I could be faced with what is essentially a page one rewrite because they think so much is very, very wrong with this draft. Yeah, I'm lucky that didn't happen.

Sob!

Heh!

ON THE FLOOR

nother radiotherapy session...
R11/19
Then...

I passed out in the bathroom this evening.

One second I was at the sink, rinsing anti-septic mouth-wash over my ulcers and, the next, BANG! On the floor.

All of which made for a rotten ending to a terrible day.

My throat is now completely burned away inside. The salivary glands and taste-buds are gone and the soft tissue is just a wall of ulcers. The only way I can swallow is by spraying artificial saliva into the back of my throat (yep, you heard...) but, even then, it's agony.

My tongue is covered in blisters, my neck is stiff and the skin on my lips is peeling away nicely.

Nice, huh?

As a result, I finally had to admit that I can no longer eat via my mouth. I'd known this was a possibility ever since I'd had the stomach peg fitted but, I'll be honest, part of me just didn't believe it would get that far.

Kirsty made me a bowl of very runny *Ready Brek* this morning, but I may as well have been trying to eat a selection of the finest scorpion arseholes. I just couldn't do it.

So, I unclipped by peg, filled it with nutrient-rich milk-shake, and breakfast was served...

...and that will also be every other meal for the next four weeks, at least.

My radiotherapy session went as well as could be expected, although I did feel a little light-headed after I came out. Lack of sleep and no real food for days. Had to be. I'd be fine after a rest.

But, things took a turn for the worse when Kirsty and I arrived home. I went for a lie down, and had just got into bed when a whole new brand of side-effect dropped in to say hello.

My throat muscles and windpipe went into spasm, flooding my chest, neck and head with sharp, shooting pains.

For a brief second, I genuinely thought I was having a heart attack. That I'd suffered some kind of bizarre reaction to today's RT session and was now paying the price.

I thought I was going to die.

It took Kirsty a good twenty minutes to calm my resulting tear-stained panic attack and, even then, she kept her finger hovering over the phone's '9' button until the pain began to subside.

I did manage to get a nap for an hour or so after that, then it was up and at 'em to pour another couple of milk-shakes down my tube. After which, I went to the bathroom to brush my teeth and rinse my mouth, and...

...well, we're back at the very start of this post again

I'm feeling down tonight, which I think is damn well allowed. I did go to bed earlier to read for a while, but have just got up to pour some liquid painkillers and yet another

300ml of laxative ('cos, that's not happened yet, either!) in via my insert pipe.

Then, I'm going back to bed.

ZZZZZZ!

Apologies for the radio silence these past few days. Tuesday's radiotherapy...

R12/18

...and Wednesday's chemo and radiotherapy...

C3/3, R13/17

...completely wiped me out.

I tried to write a couple of blog posts after returning home, but I was so drained I simply had to head straight to bed. Besides, the only thing I could think of to write about were the ins and outs of artificial saliva - but using the stuff turns my stomach.

No, thinking about the stuff turns my stomach, using the stuff causes the contents of said stomach to spot a vague glimmer of hope for escape the wrong way down my peg.

I just couldn't do it to you!

The postman brought something rather lovely today - a *Scream Street* card and a gift from the wonderful people at *Walker Books* - on the front of which, *Resus* has appeared to morphed into me!

Thanks so much to everyone at Walker Books for their kind thoughts and messages!

Yesterday's chemo session was a nightmare! The first bad experience since I first started with them.

My nurse for the day was in charge of a side room containing a chair and a bed. I was first in for the day, so I picked the bed figuring I could always catch 40 winks if I got bored eating or watching movies on my iPad, etc.

I did more than that!

I slept fitfully for almost the entire five hours of chemo! It must have been the lack of sleep finally catching up with me. I didn't intend to snore the day away, but I was zonked!

Fair enough, you might think - you need the sleep, you take it. But the set up for the day wasn't easy. It took four tries to get my cannula in, after which a nurse brought up the prospect of putting another temporary line into my body.

This one would be a cannula which the doctors would use to draw blood and feed in my chemo drugs from now on. It would fit under my left arm and stay there until my treatment was completely over.

OK...

Keep talking...

Then she pulled out a prosthetic arm to show me how the line they fed in wouldn't just go under my skin. In fact, it would connect to a longer tube which would travel across my chest, then turn down to reach my heart, and-

Wait a minute! This would lead directly into my heart?!

Yes, of course.

I'll struggle on with the regular cannulas. Thank you.

At another point during the day, the doctor came to see me to check up on how I was coping with my pain medication. She seemed to think I was taking too much at intervals that are spaced too far apart - so, today I've started taking fewer doses, but more regularly.

Gripping stuff! I'll keep you updated on how it goes.

Today's radiotherapy session...

R14/16

...went smoothly enough - although it didn't help the brand new batch of ulcers that have erupted along the sides of my tongue as a result of yesterday's chemo.

There was a brief discussion as to whether I would need to have a new mask fitted as I'm still losing weight, and the original isn't quite as tight nor snugging as once it was. But, in the end, the radiographers decided to continue with this mask for another week and take a look at it then.

So, tomorrow I reach the end of week three. The mid-way point in my cancer treatment. In some ways the time has just flown by, whereas in others...

Finally, I received a card today from Alec, aged 7, that shows me literally kicking cancer's butt!

Thanks Alec!

I Don't Do 'No'

So, I'm now three weeks through my cancer treatment...

R15/15, C3/3

Half way.

And I feel dreadful. I really do. I'd like to be able to offer some words of comfort for anyone else who is having to go through this and say that it won't be as bad as everyone promises, but I just can't do that.

It's horrible.

On top of the side-effects previously mentioned, I'm now spitting up gobs of yellow/brown stringy goo - the result, I'm led to believe, of no longer producing saliva.

It's disgusting, and has rendered me almost mute. I can't open my mouth to talk without looking like an extra from a bad zombie movie.

And I've got another three weeks of this shit to come.

Which is why I'm not celebrating this milestone at all.

Other people are - Kirsty, the boys, well-wishers, etc. But, all I can think of 'if this is what it's like after week three, what will I feel like after week five, or six?'

I'm dreading it.

Really dreading it.

But that doesn't mean I'm giving up.

It's not the same.

I was visited by the nutritionist on Friday, who happened to mention that I've reached the stage where a lot of people give up on their treatment. They simply say 'no more', and walk away.

Well, what she actually said was that they 'lose' a lot of patients at this stage of the treatment, then hastily corrected herself when she saw the expression of horror wash over my face.

But, I can't imagine doing that, no matter how much the idea of never going back appeals to me. I've started down this path, and I'll get to the end of it.

I've never been one for giving up.

Quite the opposite.

I was four years old when I decided I wanted to be on stage.

I remember the moment quite clearly...

I was at the wedding of my Dad's brother Les, to his new bride, Lyn. I sat at the reception, listening to the band play and seeing how much fun everyone was getting out of what they were playing and singing.

I wanted some of that for myself!

So, at the end of the next song, I approached the guy at the front and asked if I could sing with them (as you would).

Three minutes and one rousing rendition of *On Mother Kelly's Doorstep* later, I got my first round of applause. And that was it.

From then on, if I spotted something that I wanted to do

- something I thought I'd be good at doing - I went for it hook, line and sinker.

School plays, drama clubs, weekend retreats... I got into them all way before the prescribed age level and worked hard until I got better and better roles.

Then came the world of work...

I left college early to take up a position as a Bluecoat at *Pontins* on the Isle of Wight. This was in the company's heyday of the mid-80s, when they had 23 different holiday parks open, and a job there was still seen as a potential stepping-stone into the entertainment business.

I spent two weeks as a general 'Blue', then was asked to move to run the children's side of the programme as 'Uncle Tommy'!

No, it didn't sound quite that bad in 1986...

After two years on the Isle of Wight, I moved to run the kids' programme at *Pontins Barton Hall* in Torquay for another two. Then, I set my sights a little further afield.

The world of cruise liners.

The way I saw it, cruise liners were floating holiday parks. It couldn't be much of a jump to move from one to the other. So, I went down to the travel agents, picked up a handful of brochures and wrote in to the companies I liked the look of. They must all need a good children's entertainers like me.

One of them - *CTC Cruise lines* - ran cruises to both the Caribbean and Russia in the same year. I really liked the sound of them.

But, they wrote back to say they didn't employ a children's entertainer on board any of their ships.

So, I wrote back, saying that they should.

And I created a mini-programme of events to show just how much fun younger passengers would have if I was there to run things.

Following a trip to London for an interview, I started work on board the *MV Kareliya* in February 1991.

I travelled the world - including extended cruises down the Amazon River, circumnavigating Africa, and to the far north of Scandinavia to witness the midnight sun (as well as those trips to Russia and the Caribbean).

I met some wonderful people and brilliant entertainers - many of whom I'm thrilled to say I'm still in touch with today! The hilariously musical *Kimika* (Nick and Tina), Steve Wright (puppets), Martin Brand (vocalist), Tom and Deese Bell as *Rainbow Cascade* (magicians), Dave Derek (band leader), a whole stable-full of dancers and many more.

Eventually, I was promoted to on-board Entertainments Manager, staying until the company had a change of policy where the entertainment was concerned - then it was time to find something new.

A role which I spotted from the dress circle.

I went along with my Mum and Dad to see *Buddy: The Buddy Holly Story* at the Empire Theatre in Liverpool. It was a fantastic show, charting the life of one of the founding fathers of rock 'n' roll.

The culmination of the show is a 45 minute recreation of Buddy's last concert, on the night he was destined to die with The Big Bopper and Ritchie Valens.

But, that wasn't what interested me most.

Before the concert, the curtain was dropped and a character called the Clearlake MC came out to warm-up the audience while the concert set was built, out of sight.

I was gobsmacked.

It was as though they'd written a part just for me!

I wrote to the producers when I got home. A few weeks later, I was standing on the stage of the *Victoria Palace Theatre* in London, a guitar strung around my neck, ready to audition...

...for a completely different part.

They were auditioning me for the role of Murray Deutch - Buddy's New York music promoter (the actor of which also understudied The Big Bopper).

But, that wasn't what I wanted.

And I knew I'd only be standing on that stage one time.

So, I told the director, Paul Mills, who was auditioning me...

ME: "Excuse me?"

PAUL: "Yes?"

ME: "This isn't the part I'd like to audition for..."

Brief silence.

PAUL: "What?"

ME: "This is Murray Deutch."

PAUL: "Yes."

ME: "I'd like to audition for the Clearlake MC."

More silence.

PAUL: "Why?"

ME: "I'd rather show you than tell you..."

Rifling of papers, whispering, pencil scratches.

PAUL: "Can someone go and get him an MC script?"

A script was passed up to the stage, and I went for it.

Gave it all I got.

I played the MC in Buddy for a total of eight years, first at the *Victoria Palace Theatre*, and then the *Strand Theatre* in the West End. I also enjoyed six months on the national UK tour, and just under three months in the show at the *Princess of Wales Theatre* in Toronto.

Once again, I'm delighted to still be in touch with so many amazing people from that time - including Paul Mills, the brilliant and wise director who reluctantly agreed to let me audition for the part I wanted!

Buddy closed in March 2002, the result of falling box-office figures following the tragedy of 9/11 a few months earlier. The show still goes out on the road to tour from time to time, and I highly recommend you see it if you can.

As for me, I went into children's theatre - moving to the north east of England where I met Kirsty - and then finally quitting the day job to write full time on 30th September 2006.

I've been at that for just under ten years now.

Which is why I'm not giving in with my treatment. As much as I'd love just to crawl back into bed for a week and hide myself away right now, I won't do it.

The battle continues.

Heads up cancer. Round four.

THAT'S LIFE

Week four has begun, with...
R16/14
It went as well as can be expected, after which I saw my consultant, Dr Biswas. As ever, he was straight down the line, explaining that while this coming week may not be entirely dreadful, that week's five and six are going to be a nightmare.

So, there's something to look forward to.

Writing about my time working on cruise liners yesterday reminded me of one of the most incredible situations I've ever found myself in. A time when I was a tiny cog in a big machine working hard to save someone's life.

We were in the midst of a cruise to the Caribbean, and had just left Jamaica after a day in port. That was my one and only trip to the island, which I remember mainly for the fact that each bus of passengers heading off for a day of sight-seeing from the ship had an armed guard on board.

For some reason, this thrilled the passengers beyond belief.

We left port at around 6pm but, just an hour later, one

of the passengers fell ill. He had internal bleeding, and we had to get him back to land and to a hospital as soon as possible.

Not an easy task.

Another ship had already taken our berth in Jamaica, meaning we couldn't simply turn around and off-load the patient.

So, as the evening progressed, the ship's purser sat in the radio room, calling out to each of the tiny islands we passed if anyone had room for the ship to dock so we could land the sick man.

No-one had space.

There had been a party on the rear deck of the ship a few days earlier, and the entertainments team had spent hours tying long palm fronds to the railings to give the place a Caribbean feel.

But, as the hour grew later and the passenger became sicker, it didn't feel like a party any more.

Of course, sometimes passengers don't make it all the way through a cruise - particularly on some of the longer itineraries where the average age of those on board errs towards triple figures (often seemingly more).

On those sad occasions, there is space available to - ahem - accommodate the less fortunate until we arrived back in the UK.

On one cruise we lost so many that the whisper in the dining room was "Don't eat the ice cream, we're not sure who's in there with it."

But, we were determined it wasn't going to happen this time.

As I may have mentioned before, the ship I worked on for the majority of my time at sea - *MV Kareliya* - was run by a Russian and Ukrainian crew, with British passengers and entertainers.

By now, crew members were lining up to donate blood to help this poor guy.

But, that wasn't a permanent solution.

We had to find a way to get him to hospital.

Then, in the early hours of the morning, an unexpected message came through on the radio. It was from a US aircraft carrier running manoeuvres in the area, and they'd heard our calls to local islands for help.

They were sending a helicopter.

They asked the captain to slow the ship down to a rate of 10 knots, and for the crew to clear everything off the back deck. An emergency alert was sent out around the crew quarters and - within minutes - deckchairs, tables, parasols and just about everything else was being hauled away into the nearest bar.

All the expensive palm fronds were cut off the railings and tossed overboard.

Then we all went outside and waited.

I stood with the man's wife (I wish I could remember his name) as the distant sound of rotor blades grew louder and louder - and then, there it was - a vast US air force helicopter, drawing in to hover over our beck deck while the ship was still moving.

Two airmen - both in their early 20s - winched down onto the deck and secured the passenger's stretcher to their equipment while the ship's doctor handed over his notes.

Then, as quickly as they had arrived, the patient was hauled up into the chopper, the airmen followed, and the aircraft banked away into the darkness.

They took the man directly to hospital in Cuba.

We spent the rest of the night celebrating with one or two (or more) vodkas out in the warm night, enjoying the bewildered looks of passengers when they got up at breakfast to secure their sun loungers for the day - only to find that they had all mysteriously disappeared!

Sadly, we later heard that the passenger didn't make it. He'd been too ill.

But, we'd tried.

And, I'd seen the best in people. People working together to help each other just because they couldn't sit by and not do anything.

People who cared.

What any of this has to do with my treatment, I'm not really certain...

...although, maybe I am.

I'm sure this memory hasn't presented itself just because I wrote about my time at sea yesterday. It's also because - for the past few months - I've been looked after by some wonderful people. Doctors, nurses, radiographers - all working as hard as possible to look after other people.

Sick, often scared people, just like me.

I'll never be able to thank them enough.

LOOOOOONG DAY

Chemo Wednesday again - and today was a looooong day!

Let's get the stats out of the way: I'm now midway through my fourth week (of six) of treatment. Side effects have hit home. I haven't eaten anything by mouth for almost two weeks. And I've driven just over 1,100 miles to and from Preston for my sessions.

C4/2, R18/12

Except I nearly didn't receive today's chemo.

I've been feeling so ill that I've spent the past two days in bed, getting up only to drive to Preston to act as a sitting (well, lying) target while Britain's finest radiographers presumable play *Radiographer Super-Galactic Blastoids* against my stubborn cancer bits.

Nausea plus fatigue equals, well... nothing really.

Just staying in bed.

Yesterday I was due in at 11.15am, but simply couldn't get up. So, Kirsty called the hospital and rearranged my session for 7pm, so that I could spend the day recuperating.

I got up at 6pm, still barely able to move. Another call. 'We're open until 9pm, but he HAS to be here today'.

Due to sheer force of will, I got there and had my RT session at 7.45pm.

But, that was it. My time driving myself to and from my appointments was at an end.

Now, I know what some of you are thinking... 'Hey we haven't seen a picture of Tommy in a ridiculous hat recently!'

Well, tough.

Because the rest of you are thinking: 'Why the hell are you driving yourself to and from hospital, you utter buffoon?!'

Because I wanted one thing I could still do for myself. One thing that I had control over. I can't even eat for flip's sake. Let me have a bit of a pootle in my car once a day!

Oh, and Kirsty can't drive.

Although you wouldn't think that with the frequent which-lane-to-be-in and watch-that-guy-over-there tips that issue forth. But that's another story...

So, today I have surrendered and asked friends and family for help with lifts to and from my hospital appointments. And I was utterly overwhelmed by the response. So many people offered that I had the entire two and a half weeks filled within an hour.

Thank you all, so much.

But, today I did drive in for chemo which, as I said, I almost didn't get.

Cancer had clearly been fighting back. And I looked so ill by the time I arrived at the ward that the nurses insisted on me being seen by a doctor before they would issue the meds. For a while, they weren't sure if I could handle any more chemo.

That sounds scary, but I've met one or two people at the *Rosemere Centre* who have been in that position. Chemo has had such a negative impact on their health that they've been forced to stop treatment.

Was I about to become one of those patients?

No.

No, I wasn't.

(Sorry. I should have built the tension up a bit more there).

The doctor arrived, checked the results of my blood tests (worryingly low in some areas), examined me and my vitals - and said I was good to go.

So, I goed. Sorry, went.

I was hooked up to my first two-hour flush and meds, and then had to wait for my black bag o' doom to arrive for the actual nasty stuff to be pumped into my body.

Except, they don't start preparing your meds until they get the go ahead from the ward, and that request came late today.

Which added another two hours onto the session.

At 5pm, I staggered out of the chemo ward and went downstairs for my radiotherapy session.

I was utterly wiped out.

This couldn't end quick enough.

I just wanted to go home.

And then there was a problem with my radiotherapy mask.

Remember that thing?

The mask has to fit tightly across my head and neck to keep me in exactly the right position for *Radiographer Super-Galactic Blastoids* (my RT).

And I've lost weight.

Quite a lot of weight.

Hurray!

But that's a bad thing here.

Boo!

The mask was now as loose, and it wasn't keeping me in the correct position.

So, it took two refits to get it right before it was blasting time.

I finally arrived home at 8pm, had two vanilla milkshakes through my stomach peg for tea (yum!), then went to bed.

Do you know...

The more I go through this cancer thing, the less I like it.

HOT RUBBER FACE HUGGER

My last day of driving to treatment (or pretty much anywhere) today, so I made sure to arrive in plenty of time for my radiotherapy session...

R19/11

Once that was completed, the radiographers explained that - because I've lost so much weight in the past four weeks - I would have to have a new mask made, and then the final two weeks of RT treatment would have to be replotted from scratch.

And they were going to do that now.

So, I had another cannula fitted (when the nurse could find a vein), and I was led to the CT scan room. I laid back on the bench, and the team soaked and brought over another flat piece of mesh.

This was then pressed down over my face and neck and moulded into place.

And it's an experience I can't really describe...

It's like having a hot rubber face hugger water-board you.

Many congrats to my good pal, Bev, for brilliantly

suggesting that *Hot Rubber Face Hugger* sounds like the title of a Frank Zappa album!

I then had to lie perfectly still for 20 minutes while the team wafted me dry with bits of card.

My life is so weird right now.

When the mask had set, I required a new CT scan so that my consultant could get straight to work plotting the final ten sessions of *Radiographer Super-Galactic Blastoids*. So, I had a contracting dye pumped in through the cannula.

And that's a strange sensation, too.

Imagine having a hot flush, a dry mouth and desperately needing a wee - all at once.

Then you'd be close.

Oh, and the nurses draw green marks on your face to help guide the lasers that line everything up. They seemed quite excited that they'd been given a brand new pen to do just this.

Until it wouldn't wipe off afterwards.

So, with a vaguely damp head covered with green stripes, Kirsty and I set off for home - and another very early night.

From tomorrow, I'm having to request lifts to and from treatment. So many people have offered their help, and I'm very, very grateful. What these wonderful people are doing is amazing, for two reasons...

It's a long journey, and Kirsty is a chatterbox. ;)

The fab George Kirk will be running me tomorrow, and for the final two Fridays.

As for me - I've got a couple of milkshakes to put down a rubber tube, then I'm off to bed. Strawberry, this time.

The milkshakes I mean. Not the bed.

One or two folk have been asking why the nutrient milkshakes are flavoured when they go in directly via the peg...

Well, they can be taken by mouth if you're still able to

swallow (which I'm not). And then there's the problem of burping.

Trust me. You want a bit of flavour when it comes to backdraft.

FEEL THE FOURTH

Today's radiotherapy session...
R20/10

I am now at the end of my fourth week of treatment.

And I feel a lot more positive about things than I did at this point last week. Yes, the final two weeks are promising to be the worst of the lot - but there is now an end in sight.

And that's what I'm aiming for.

After which, the tricky business of recuperation begins.

I'm told that, for the first two weeks post treatment my side effects will remain, and possibly worsen. But, after that, I should be on the up and up each day.

I can't wait!

Nor can I wait to enjoy some proper food again.

Just because I can't eat doesn't mean I don't want to.

I've started staying in my office while the family eats together. Not because I don't want to be downstairs with them, but it just depresses me! They're having chicken this evening. Chicken with potatoes and vegetables.

Insert Homer Simpson drooling sound effect.

I've got caramel milkshakes on the menu tonight. Not that I'll taste them at all.

Kirsty has decided to get me a NutriBullet, so that we can experiment with making fruit and vegetable juices that can be administered via the peg. It's another way of taking vitamins and minerals on board - and may not make me feel quite so sickly as the milkshakes do.

I want cheese and crackers.

I love cheese and crackers.

Sigh.

Many, many thanks to the awesome George Kirk for running me to hospital and back today - a trip during which she encountered a sudden tyre pressure alert while on the M65 and, spookily, while explaining about the last time this had happened.

While I was being blasted with invisible health, George nipped to a nearby garage to get it checked out. Thankfully, it turned out to just be a switch that needed resetting.

My brilliant sister, Sue, is on driving duty for Monday, Tuesday and Wednesday next week, followed by my good pal, Alison, on Thursday and George again on Friday.

I really can't thank everyone enough.

And I really have to thank Isaac and Stanley for the amazing image they sent me! They are the sons of Rachel, one of the nurses who looks after me on the chemo ward. It turns out they're big fans of Scream Street on TV, so I took a couple of books in for them last week.

Now comes the weekend. Lots of rest is planned for yours truly, and I plan to crack on with the rewrite of my new book. It will be a great way to take my mind off more troubling matters, and have fun in the process!

HAIR-LUCINATIONS

So, here we go with week five of my treatment.

Just this week and next to go.

In some ways, it has flown by. In others, not so much.

One thing that has flown, however, is my hair. When I was first diagnosed, I was told that I probably wouldn't lose it all - perhaps just a bit at the back where the super whizzo magic beams pierce my supple, alabaster flesh in search of cancer orcs to battle (I'm pretty sure that's scientifically correct).

And, that's more or less exactly what has happened.

Although the back and sides have now almost disappeared.

Unless I wanted to look like an extra from the first series of *The Black Adder*, something needed to be done.

My sister, Sue, in addition to running me to hospital and back today, brought her clippers along and shaved it (almost) all off. I still have a fine fuzz there to keep the shine off.

It's certainly a new look for me.

I quite like it.

But now I look like I've got cancer.

Either that or I'm just not wearing my Doc Martens, Union Jack t-shirt and braces, or walking my badly trained pit bull (who is probably called something like Killer or Mauler or Bastard or, I dunno... Simon).

When 9yo Sam got home from school, he spent a good ten minutes just rubbing my head. Then he said I look like I'm 70 years old, and went upstairs to fire up his PlayStation.

Kids.

SAM

What can I say about my son, Sam?

He. Is. Amazing!

Sam's life started on a very quiet note. He was born asleep.

Yes, you read that correctly. He was born asleep.

At first, the lack of crying or any other noise concerned Kirsty and I, and we asked if everything was OK with him.

"Oh yes," came the reply. "We're just trying to wake him up!"

I can't think of a better way to introduce Sam to you.

As he grew, we became aware that he was someone special. Even as young as three or four months, as he lay in his little blue bouncy chair, he started to pay attention to the most unexpected things. The main one being the TV show, *QI*. We knew, of course, that he was too young to understand what he was watching (not that we sat him in front of the television especially, of course). It has always been one of my favourite programmes and, whenever I tuned in to watch it, he would sit, absolutely absorbed, in a way that he didn't display with any other TV show, even those we showed him that were made especially for children his age.

As he developed, we noticed that he had an aversion to loud noises, and that he flapped his hands whenever he was happy or excited. This continued as he grew, leading us to suspect that he may possibly have Asperger's Syndrome - a form of autism.

This was confirmed at the end of his first year at school. Although he would staying in the same class as he moved from Reception to Year 1, the day the teachers removed the wall displays and prepared the classroom in readiness for the new school year starting in September affected him badly. He simply couldn't cope with the change, and that's when we knew.

However, it is not true to say that Sam in any way *suffers* from Asperger's. If anything, he thrives because of it. This is what's known as high-functioning Asperger's. As a result, Sam is incredibly smart, devours facts, figures and any kind of new information, and shows an incredible level of interest in any topic he begins to enjoy.

The biggest of these is penguins. Sam adores them, and constantly teaches himself everything he can about the animals. At the age of four or five, he could reel off the names of all the different breeds, which part of the world they lived in, and what made them different from their similar cousins.

It was around this time that he announced to the family that he wanted to be a penguinologist when he grew up. Yeah, I had to look it up, as well. It is, as you might deduce, a marine biologist who specialises in the research and care of penguins. Since then, he has plotted his entire career path, looking up college and university courses, qualifications, and everything else he will need to learn about in order to achieve his goal.

You may remember that, at the same age, I announced to

my own parents that I wanted to be an actor. That, along with many, many other similarities have led me to believe that I also have Asperger's, and always have had.

We call ourselves The Aspie Boys.

Sam's favourite toy was and still is a teddy penguin his Uncle Les and Aunt Lyn bought him for his very first Christmas. His name is PayPay, and he goes everywhere with Sam, staying in the car when he goes into school so that he's there waiting for him when he comes back out at the end of the day.

He showed an aptitude for technology at a very early age, picking up Kirsty's computer and teaching himself to use it - and not just to play games. So, we picked him up a second hand laptop, set the parental controls, and let him loose.

I recall one day when I was writing in my office, and Sam - then aged around 4 - popped in to ask if he could borrow "my dedit card".

I asked if he meant 'debit card', and he confirmed that he did, but wouldn't elaborate further as to why he needed it. So, I followed him back into his bedroom where, on his laptop screen, I saw that he had been trying to book the family a holiday to Disneyland! He'd chosen dates, filled in all of our names, and got as far as the checkout page when he was forced to stop. He had attempted to invent a string of numbers to use for payment purposes and, when they hadn't worked, had decided to simply ask me for the use of my card.

We kept a very close eye on him after that!

His computing skills continued to flourish, and he did everything from watch videos on how film makers mix together fake blood for their movies, to teaching himself the basics of programming and, at the present time, shooting and editing his own videos for his own YouTube channel.

His latest project has been to modify some of his

favourite computer console games so that he can add extra characters, locations, sound effects and more.

There are now times when he shows Kirsty and I how to achieve what we're trying to get done online.

He obviously does well at school, although this is where he occasionally has problems due to a lack of expertise in social skills. Early on, he would announce that he didn't want to work with certain other pupils as they were stupid, and would slow him down. He became very upset and apologetic when it was explained to him that his comments were hurtful, and he's getting better at holding his tongue as time passes. At least until he gets home and can vent his frustrations in private.

Rarely a day goes by when Sam doesn't do something to surprise me - from the time he offered to sing nursery rhymes for his Granddad, charging him a pound per song *after* he'd performed the first two, to entering his school talent show as a stand up comedian - writing, rehearsing and then performing his own five-minute routine.

Unfortunately, Sam has been very badly affected by my battle with cancer. While Arran simply doesn't talk about it, Sam worries that the worst is going to happen.

We frequently have tears before school - something that has never happened before - and he often asks to have his temperature checked when he gets up, because he wants us to tell him he's ill and can stay at home with me.

No matter how many times Kirsty and I explain to him that I'm getting better, and that I'm now dealing with the side effects of my treatment rather than the cancer itself, he remains terrified that I'm going to collapse at any moment.

We took him along to one of my hospital appointments so that my oncologist could explain the details to him. Dr Biswas was wonderful and answered all of his questions, but it made very little difference.

A few evenings back, he came down from his room physically shaking and in floods of tears. He threw his arms around me and wouldn't let go. When he'd finally calmed down enough to speak, he said, "Dad, I don't want you to die the same way as Granddad."

A night or two later, he started to panic because I was dancing gently to some music (my only form of exercise and prescribed by the doctors to get me moving around. I may look daft, but it helps!) He was scared I was going to fall and be rushed into intensive care again. In the end I had to dance next the couch so he could hold my hand.

We're working hard with his school teachers to ensure that he is able to come to terms with my illness, and he has just started to receive visits from a specialist counsellor who is trained to help children in this situation.

I feel terrible for being the cause of Sam's distress, however unintentionally, and love the moments when he forgets about his concerns and goes back to being his usual, brilliant self.

He's the light of my life, and one of the reasons I will continue to fight this dreadful disease with every ounce of my strength.

Watch out for Sam Donbavand - he's going to make his mark on this world.

TEN

As mentioned in my previous post, today was the start of my fifth week of cancer treatment. Two weeks - just ten days to go.

Today's session was...

R21/9

...and it was unusual. The radiographers aren't using my new mask yet, but someone seems to have tried to tighten up my old one for use in the meantime.

Either that, or my head has grown over the weekend.

The result was that my face was squashed painfully flat whenever the team tried to secure my mask to the bench.

Ow!

After some fiddling around, they had to slide out a layer of supports from the headrest so that they could clip the mask in place without straining me through the meshed material like mashed potato.

Still, we got there in the end.

A scan, and regular radiotherapy followed.

After which, I waited to see my consultant, Dr Biswas. He had nipped off to take a look at the results of today's scan.

He came back smiling.

It was good news.

He was delighted with the scan.

He said that if he'd known five weeks ago that I would be doing so well at this stage, he would have been very happy indeed.

He even offered to cancel my final two chemo sessions, saying they would now be just a tiny part of the battle. I gratefully refused.

Best to get as much cancer kicking in as I can while I can, I reckon.

Now - this is NOT the all clear.

I'm NOT in remission. I'm NOT cured.

But the treatment is working!

The effects of the radiotherapy will continue for at least two weeks after I stop being zapped by wonderful people in white coats.

After that, everything inside has to heal and repair before I can go back for tests to see what's what.

For the first time in many, many weeks - I feel a faint glimmer of optimism.

NINE

I'm now well into the single figure countdown for my radiotherapy treatment today with session...

R22/8

Just eight more sessions to go.

I hope they're not all like today's.

I was warned that the final two weeks would be the hardest to handle, and that's already looking as though it will be the case. I didn't sleep much last night thanks to the pain of new ulcers and a slowly tightening constriction down the inside of my throat.

I was in a lot of pain.

A promised, it feels like sunburn on the inside.

If I didn't know any better, I might say the cancer was making a last stand.

Maybe I don't know better...

But... OW!

What little sleep I did get was punctuated by dealing with the copious amounts of gunk my throat now seems keen - if not eager - to produce. It's horrible, horrible stuff - and the part of this process I will miss the least.

Plus, I'm now kicking myself for not buying shares in paper kitchen towels before over half of our weekly shopping trolley was taken up by dozens of rolls of the stuff.

My sister ran me to hospital and back again yesterday. Which is just as well, as I spent most of the journey nodding off. I came close to sleep once or twice under the scanner/blaster, too.

In fact, I probably would have had to be woken by the radiographers if, you know, I hadn't been battling an incurable illness for, at best, my ability to speak and, at worst, my life.

Trust me, that's a thought that will keep you awake. Especially with the dulcet tones of the Cancer Killer 9000 revolving around your tightly-pinned meshed head.

It wasn't all doom and gloom, however. I waited in the usual waiting area for the treatment and - as ever - one of the radiographers opened the door to an unoccupied changing cubicle and called me over...

"Tommy!"

As I headed in his direction, I could see that he was grinning. And then he added...

"Or, should I call you B. Strange?"

B. Strange! I haven't been called that name in years! Back when I was starting out as a full time writer, I was hired by Egmont Press to write five books in a new kids' comedy horror series called Too Ghoul For School.

As there were several of us working on the series, the publisher came up with a spooky sounding name for the 'author'.

B. Strange.

I think I've been outed!

By the time I got home, I was so exhausted that all I could do was crawl into bed and sleep for a couple of hours.

Until today's particular side effects found their own, shrilling voice, that was.

I can't say I'm looking forward to tomorrow. A full day of chemo, followed by another session under the bug zapper of death.

'Til then...

EIGHT

Another looooong day!
The good bit - sessions...
C5/1, R23/7
...are done and dusted, baby!
Seven days of treatment to go.

Hurray!

The not so good bit...

My sister ran me to the chemo ward this morning, although I can't say I was particularly chatty during the journey. I had another dreadful night last night with a combination of throat and mouth pain, and the seemingly unstoppable tsunami of gooey crap that wants to issue forth.

I can't wait for this to be over.

It's starting to get me down and, as I'm spending much of the night up and alone, I don't want the dark thoughts to start circling again like birds of prey.

Evil, nasty birds of prey with cold, dark eyes and sharp beaks.

And excellent excrement targeting abilities.

I'll have to be careful.

Anyhoo...

Many of you may know that finding a vein in which to insert a cannula isn't exactly an easy process where I'm concerned. And, of course, chemo can't begin until that has happened.

Today was the worst of the lot. Several attempts in - including one that stung like a Nazi wasp licking acid from a thistle - and a plan was concocted.

NURSE: "We need to heat your hands."

ME: "Sorry?"

NURSE: "Your hands. If we heat them, it can sometimes help the veins to raise up and show themselves."

ME: "Oh, OK. How do we do that, then?"

They gave me a pair of electronically heated mittens to wear.

I sat for twenty minutes looking like an albino Pingu while the nurses hurried off to deal with other patients and left me to bake slowly under a medium heat from the fingers down.

But, it did the trick and - half an hour later - I was all cannulad up and ready to go. My first bags of fluid - anti-sickness drugs and detoxing flush - were set up...

...and I fell straight to sleep.

In fact, I dozed in fits and starts for most of the day.

I had hoped to get some work done, but they'd only been able to connect the chemo to my right hand, which meant that had to stay perfectly still.

Ah well.

Fast forward five long hours, and I was free to go. Well, to go downstairs and have my radiotherapy session. I was on a machine in a different lab for that today, although I'd met two of the three radiographers there before.

Gripping stuff this blog, isn't it?

Finally, my sister ran me home where I now sit - staring at

the two lovely yummy disgusting sickly bottle of nutrient-rich vanilla milkshake that I know I have to flush down my tube before I do much else.

Sigh.

Although... Kirsty got me a NutriBullet this week. She's going to make some high energy juices for the peg (and eventually, my mouth) to make sure I continue taking all the right vitamins and minerals on board.

In the meantime, I'm off for a lie down where I imagine I'll dream of myself as the Vanilla Ice of the penguin world...

SEVEN

I've just returned from today's radiotherapy session...

R24/6

Six sessions left to go.

And it can't go quickly enough as far as I'm concerned.

I'm so, so tired.

Plus, the side effects are now stacking on top of each other to cause me problems - like seven angry squirrels on each other's shoulders inside a buttoned-up raincoat.

The outside of my neck is red, hot and painful to the touch. Being the ginger variety of human, sunburn has always been part of my life - usually followed by bouts of heat-stroke induced soaring temperatures where I hallucinate that I'm zooming between the corners of the bedroom ceiling in one of two racing cars (I want the yellow car, not the red one!)

This feels just like sunburn. No Formula One level fever yet, but I'll have to keep an eye on that as once I hit 38 degrees, that's me being admitted to hospital (chemo rules).

The inside of my throat is now almost completely constricted, and swallowing is pure agony.

Even sips of water feel like daggers.

But, I HAVE to keep trying. If I don't, I've been told I could lose my reflux completely - and with that finally goes the voice. Cue weeks of speech and swallowing therapy to be added to the end of this malarkey.

I really don't want that to happen.

And then, there are the ulcers.

Be pleased, dear reader, that I can't speak well at the moment and therefore I am typing this blog post, rather than using any form of dictation system.

For that would have picked up the name I just called those ulcers, and most of you would now be running for the hills, horrified that a gentle, caring children's author could even know of such a word, let alone scream it out loud.

As for the rest of you - those with sterner stomachs and minds of experience - you'd probably just be wondering how much you would have a pay the gorilla just to wear something like that, never mind operate the mincer blades.

In short: the ulcers hurt.

A lot.

And the constant mucus...

Which - today - comes with a free gift of blood every single time I cough!

Cancer. The disease that keeps on giving.

However, the day wasn't a complete waste. My good friend Alison was kind enough to take me to hospital today.

Alison and I have known each other for years. In fact, since the day we both joined the cast of *Buddy: The Buddy Holly Story* in London's glitzy West End.

May 1994, if I recall correctly.

I'd just been summoned to the wardrobe department of the Victoria Palace Theatre to be fitted for my Clearlake MC costume, arriving just as Alison (although I didn't know her name then) was getting re-dressed after her appointment.

"Oh, hello!" she grinned. "You've just missed the good bit!"

We've been great mates ever since. We've lived together in both London and Toronto, shared tour accommodation, and attended each other's weddings.

So, that was today.

I'm utterly exhausted now, and may attempt a nap before the nutritionist is due to visit at 4pm. After which, I have some actual writing work to do this evening.

Looking forward to that!

But, for now...

ZZZZZZZZZ!

SIX

L ast night I started to write a blog post about the end of my fifth week of cancer treatment - and it's true.

Just one week left to go.

Hurray!

However, while writing, a few negative feelings which were lurking at the back of my mind hijacked the post, waved an imaginary sword around (I don't do guns, not even in my imagination), and steered the post off in a different, darker direction.

I woke up this morning planning to rewrite the post - but now I don't know if I should.

What I wrote last night came from the heart (with a quick pass by the spleen, just to make sure it was sprinkled with sourness).

If I go back and rewrite it, it will be as though I'm denying myself having had those thoughts - which I'm not.

Which I never will do on this blog.

That was genuinely how I felt last night.

I mean - come on... I've had to endure this nonsense for

five long weeks. Over 1,500 miles of motorway to get to a place where I'll struggle to park, and then people much younger and smarter than me strap me to a table and blast me with radiation!

And there's just ONE week left to go!!

Get in!

So, here's the deal...

I've added my original blog post. below. If you want to read how I was feeling last night, please continue down the page.

Don't worry, it's not that dark. I just allowed the late hour, fatigue and painful mouth ulcers get the better of me.

And I was most likely off my tits on nutrient-heavy strawberry milkshakes.

If you'd rather just revel in this bit, where I am (partially) rested, warm, fuzzy and jolly - stop right here.

Well, not right there - I've got one or two more sentences to type first.

Still with me? Good.

OK. Stop...

NOW!

Or, don't...

Written and posted in the evening of Friday 20th May...

Week five of my cancer treatment is now done and dusted!

Today's session was...

R25/5

It went smoothly enough, once we'd sorted out the tight mask issue one again. No-one seems quite sure why that is happening...

So, I have just one week of cancer treatment left to go!

Five sessions of radiotherapy, and one of chemotherapy.

My feelings on the subject are mixed. Obviously, I'll be delighted when the constant back and forth to the Royal Preston Hospital is finished with (major thanks to the lovely George Kirk for today's driving duties!)

But, everyone at the Rosemarie Cancer Foundation has been SO wonderfully kind, caring and patient that I will miss seeing them each day.

I won't miss the sessions themselves, of course - although I'm told the side effects will continue to worsen for a week or two before they subside.

So, there's that to look forward to.

Radiotherapy - the nuclear-powered invisible laser medicine that keeps on giving!

And, finally, this has got to work. Should the cancer ever return in the same place, treatment is out of the question.

I can't have radiotherapy on the right hand side of my throat and neck ever again.

If it returns elsewhere, it's a possibility. Just not the same area.

Which is nagging at me a little.

Since I was diagnosed, I've received so many lovely emails from people telling me their stories in the fight against this horrible illness, or the way their close friends and family members battled onwards.

I've heard all kinds of amazing tales: 'five years free', 'ten years and no return', 'in remission', 'cured', and many more.

But, and this is where things start to get darker, folks - so feel free to click away or tune out if you're currently enjoying some kind of fantastic Friday feeling.

There's probably something good on TV right about now...

OK, have they all gone now?

Right. Here's what I think...

I think the cancer will come back.

One day.

This is what is going to get me.

In the end.

I always suspected it would be my breathing. Asthma, chest infection, pneumonia or one of those jolly wheezing japes.

But, no. This is the thing.

Cancer.

I watched it take both of my parents and then turn around, hungry for more.

Of course, I'll be trying with all my might to stop that from happening. Once I'm well again, everything changes – choice of diet, cut out drinking (bar special occasions), regular exercise, (more) weight loss, etc.

But, that's no guarantee.

You see, cancer's had a taste of me now. And I genuinely believe it will come back, sniffing around for seconds. Maybe not for many years, but it will.

And then I have to decide whether I can go through all this again. If not for me, then for Kirsty and the boys.

I've just paused to read back what I've written so far. Not exactly uplifting stuff to be writing at the end of week five, is it?

Sorry about that.

It's just that I really can see the light at the end of the tunnel now. And part of me is scared to step out into that light...

...in case there's just another tunnel waiting dead ahead.

Does that make sense?

What worries me is that I've never felt that way about anything before. In fact, I've always relished that leap into the unknown; jumping in with both feet to see where and how I land.

Making the most of the unchartered lands ahead.

Except, I really don't want to come back here.

Not to this place.

And I'm almost convinced I will do just that.

Plus, if this is what it takes and feels in order to get well again, imagine what not getting well from this bastard must be like.

I accidentally typed that in an email to my agent the other day.

I meant to say that 'I will get well, and crack on with Project MH' (a potential new series for her to take to publishers).

But, I didn't write that.

For some unknown reason, I actually typed: 'I will not get well, and crack on...'

She made me delete the email.

But that little typo has been bugging me ever since.

Reading too much into a silly mistake? Perhaps.

Letting the black ferrets of darkness emerge from the shadows and scarper up my trouser legs? Almost certainly.

But it's there. Gnawing at my every thought.

This isn't over.

Cancer will be back.

And, when it arrives, I'll have to be ready and waiting.

Again.

FIVE

Well, my voice has finally disappeared.
As of today...
R26/4
...I can whisper hoarsely, or make wild inappropriate gestures that get across what I'm trying to say in no meaningful way whatsoever.

It's quite weird.

There's just nothing there.

Plus, I've been warned that when my voice does return, it might sound completely different.

If that's right, can I pick what I get?

A quick note out to the universe: I'd prefer James Earl Jones to Jamie Oliver.

Just saying.

Or, rather, not saying.

But my speech (or lack thereof) is not my real reason for entry.

No, that's because this is coming your way...

The #TommyVCancer Blog Tour

Organised by the incredible Vivienne Dacosta, this tour

will read and review books written by yours truly for the ENTIRE month of June - with most days featuring two separate websites!

How cool is that?!

I'm told there will be prizes to snatch up along the way (keep an eye on the tour for details as I don't have all the info - yet!)

Wow!

Just wow!

THANK YOU so much to Viv, all the bloggers and everyone who plans to follow along and read about the books I've written.

I'm overwhelmed.

FOUR

Today was...

R27/3

...and I barely made it through. I'm now very weak and tired all the time. I sleep so much, which has to be my body's way of telling me that it needs to shut down all energetic processes and focus all its attention on rebuilding the damage both the radiotherapy and chemotherapy are doing to me.

And make no mistake about it - the treatment for my cancer is not safe. Not in the slightest. There's a reason the radiographers fasten me to a bench so that I can't move, then dash to the safety of a different room to operate the vast laser machine of dooooooom (yes, six 'o's) and fire x-rays through my skin and into the soft tissue beyond. And dash, they do. They mainly confine their exits to a brisk walk, but there have been occasions when they out and out run away from the contraption I'm strapped to - like the henchmen of a Bond villain, escaping the death rays of a megalomaniac's machine of murder.

Which would make me James Bond, I guess.

Cool!

Chemotherapy, however, isn't cool. It's a system where nurses purposefully pump poisonous chemicals into my body in the hope that they will kill the bad cancer cells along with the perfectly healthy cells just going about their daily business around them. Sort of like nuking the whole of Los Angeles, just to stop Adam Sandler from making any more movies.

Wow - from James Bond to Adam Sandler in one paragraph. That's a hell of a come down.

And now all I can think about is Adam Sandler being named as the new Bond after Daniel Craig. How much would that suck?

James Bond returns in 'Please Say Never Again'

shudder

Speaking of James Bond...

After writing Scream Street, I next pitched a series to my publisher about a vampire spy, then called *Fangs Charisma*. He was to be a comedy Bond spoof, with a werewolf sidekick (the smart one of the team) named *Puppy Galore*.

There were going to be six books:

The Man With The Golden Bum

Octopixie

On Her Majesty's Supernatural Service

Dr. Nobody

Moonhowler

Trollsinger

Fangs - agent *Double O Negative* - and Puppy worked for MP1, a secret government organisation that worked to protect innocent humans from the creatures they shared the planet with. MP1 was run by *Phlem*, ably assisted by his toothless banshee secretary, *Miss FunnyGummy*. *Professor Hubert Cubit* - aka *Cube* - provided the gadgets, and *Dr Anna Nowkoff* was in charge of medical support.

I had such a blast writing the books - but the infamous

'difficult second album' influence hit hard. My publishers didn't believe that my young readers would be able to easily pronounce the word 'charisma', so Fangs' surname had to change.

I came up with HUNDREDS of alternatives, none of which could be settled on - until, over a year later, they finally agreed to one of my very first suggestions. Enigma. *Fangs Charisma* became *Fangs Enigma*.

This may sound strange to non-authors, but trying to write a novel - let alone a series of six - while not being able to pin down something as basic as your main character's name, makes life very difficult indeed.

Then, my publisher's lawyers decided that *Eon Productions*, the producers of the Bond movies, may sue due to copyright infringement. I tried to push the case for parody (as has been seen in many other projects), but it was to no avail.

The books all had to be rewritten, removing any obvious Bond gags (the codename *Double O Negative* and the character names *Puppy Galore*, and *Miss FunnyGummy* among them. Say hello to *Puppy Brown* and *Miss Bile*). Plus, all of the titles had to change, becoming...

Operation: Golden Bum
Codename: The Tickler
Assignment: Royal Rescue
Target: Nobody
Project: Wolf World
Mission: Lullaby

Not bad, but not as strong as my original ideas, in my humble opinion.

This, of course, delayed publication (something that had already happened on several other occasions) and left me with a *Scream Street* readership that had moved on to other books and authors.

As a result of all this - my *Fangs: Vampire Spy* series was a flop. No matter how much I loved the world and its characters, and how much fun I had writing the books, there was no scope for more. And that was a huge shame.

I should make a point here... I am NOT in any way blaming my publisher for the problems with *Fangs*, or its lack of success. It was simply a case of it being the wrong series at the wrong time. One of those unfortunate publishing things.

That said, the kids who have read the books LOVED them! Every year, authors receive a payment known as Public Lending Right. We pen-monkeys get around 6p every time one of our books is borrowed from a UK library (and similar systems exist in other countries). Bearing in mind that I now have over 100 books listed for PLR, my six *Fangs: Vampire Spy* books are always in the top 10 most popular books, and are frequently the top six themselves!

I'd give up my licence to kill (fictional characters) if I could write another series of adventures for Fangs and Puppy but, sadly, that looks very unlikely.

If you want to know more about the series and download samples and other goodies, you can visit the *Fangs Enigma* website at...

www.fangsvampirespy.com

THREE

Both of today's sessions went well, therein lies the tale...

Today was supposed to be my final chemo session, but I was too ill to do it. That sounds strange, I know - I was too ill to receive treatment for my illness, but it was true.

I could barely move this morning. I'd arranged for a friend to give myself and Kirsty a lift to Preston so that I could be pumped full of yummy chemicals, but I simply couldn't get out of bed.

The last time I'd seen my oncologist, Dr Biswas, he had offered to cancel my final two chemotherapy sessions, explaining that it was clear they were having an adverse effect on me, and that the chemo was around 5% of my treatment, whereas the radiotherapy made up the remaining 95% (why I'm not allowed to miss any of those sessions).

Bravely, I said 'no'. I'd promised myself - and my family - that I was going to do everything to rid myself of this malignant bastard, and that's what I was going to do, even if it caused me extreme discomfort and distress.

But that was two weeks ago. Last week's chemo session had been tough, and I'd almost crawled away from it on my hands and knees, begging for mercy.

But, this week... There was no way I was going to get through this week's appointment, at least not with the ability to exist in any meaningful way.

So, Kirsty called and spoke to Dr Biswas, accepting his offer to end my chemotherapy early. I felt really bad asking her to do it. I mean, what if this final session was the one that made all the difference? As highly unlikely as that was, it was still possible. What if I was signing my name on the dotted line of a one-way ticket to the writing room in the sky by missing out on one more period of poison pumping through my veins?

It was terrifying to think about, but not as terrifying as the prospect of being connected up to that stuff ever, ever again.

So, I missed my final chemo session, and made it (barely) to Preston in time for my radiotherapy appointment. That one wasn't negotiable.

Now, if you'll excuse me, I'm going back to bed for a decade or two.

TWO

I t's so close, I can almost taste it. (The end of my treatment, that is - not the x-rays being blasted at me). Today was...

R29/1

I never thought I'd reach this point in my treatment, especially during the past week when I've had a severe drop in energy, strength and all-round wanting to do any of this shit at all.

What's worse - and this is so much a 'first world problem' is that my last few radiotherapy sessions have been taking place in the older part of the radiography department at the *Rosemere Cancer Centre*.

I started out in the brand spanking new area - a modern, bright waiting room with comfy chairs, new treatment rooms with up-to-the-minute equipment and decor. It was like stepping into the future for my treatment.

But, further down the hall, sits the original part of the facility. The waiting room furniture is more old-fashioned, the decor less modern, and the radiotherapy equipment is older and more used. Some of it has fading paint and worn down instruction panels.

Which is a ridiculous thing to even think about. But, in my defence, when you're pinned down to a narrow bench by a mask that fits securely over your face and prevents you from moving so much as a few millimetres, you have to occupy your mind with something.

Quick side note: you are allowed to bring your favourite music along to play while you go through your radiotherapy sessions, but I warned against this by one of the cancer nurses earlier on. Why? Because she said it's easy to link the music you're listening to and the discomfort of the treatment sessions, and even the cancer - thus ruining what has been some of your favourite music for all time. At first, I didn't think that possible - but I'll explain in a later post how that became very true indeed.

So, I've been treated in the older part of the radiography department. And that doesn't matter one tiny bit. I'm only bringing it up because it's something I don't think I've talked about yet, and coming up with another topic for today's post would require a tiny bit of effort on my part - effort which I couldn't summon with a magic wand, even if I could be bothered.

Which I'm not.

Big day tomorrow. So go away.

ONE

R30/0!
Celebrate, good times - come on!
er...
Lie in bed, wiped out - come on!

That's more like it.

But, I did it! I have finished my cancer treatment. I've been through 30 consecutive radiotherapy sessions, and five out my six scheduled chemotherapy sessions.

It's finally over!

Thank the Flying Spaghetti Monster in the sky.

My sister, Sue, once again very kindly ran myself and Kirsty to Preston today, and was in the car park with her daughter, Aoife, to collect me when it was all over.

I couldn't walk properly, so Kirsty had to hold me up as I left the building. I wasn't going to leave in a wheelchair - I was going to walk out of there.

And I did, with one fist held high in the air. Triumphant.

I did it. And I never want to go through anything like that ever again.

Although, I may have to.

You may recall a post where I met an older gentleman at the *Rosemere Cancer Centre* who'd had exactly the same cancer as me, and went through an almost identical course of treatment a year ago. Then, his cancer returned - on the opposite side of his neck - and he was embarking on this awful journey for a second time.

That could happen to me.

Obviously, I really hope and pray that it doesn't, but it's a possibility.

You see, where the doctors can never give me any more radiotherapy for the right hand side of my throat - they *can* reverse the angles, and target the left side.

Which led to a very strange conversation with Kirsty once we'd arrived back at home. She asked me...

If the cancer comes back, would you go through that treatment again?

The truth? I don't know. I really don't.

I'd like to think that I'd want to blast the bugger into bits just as I hope this course of treatment has hopefully done - but, the way I'm feeling at the moment, I think I'd rather close my eyes and never open them again.

Which is a horrifying prospect.

Not for me, however.

Let me explain...

This experience has taught me a lot of things - some of which I can put into words (and have been doing), and some that I think will take me a long time to find a way to articulate, if that's possible at all.

One thing I have learned is that I'm not scared of dying - at least, not from my point of view. If I'm correct in my beliefs, I won't know anything about it at all.

The universe existed quite happily for over 13 billion years before I was alive, and will continue to do so - hopefully for billions more - when I'm no longer doing so. Just like everything else around us, I'm made of atoms, which will eventually go their separate ways in search of new adventures.

Not being alive certainly didn't bother me from the period between the Big Bang and my conception, and I presume I'll be just as blasé about it from the moment of my death until the end of time and space.

But - should I pop off to meet the great editor in the sky, it will have a profound and terrible effect on my family. Especially, Kirsty, Sam and Arran. And my brother, Bryan, and sister, Sue.

And that's what changes everything.

So what if I'm utterly shagged out by all these weeks of treatment? So what if I can barely move and speak? So what if I haven't eaten a solid meal for months on end? I'm not here for me.

Wow, that's quite a concept to take on board, isn't it? So, I'll say it again.

I'm not here for me.

I'm here for others. To make the world a better place for my family, my friends, the people around me and - ultimately - the world at large.

I'd like to think that's why we're all here: to make a difference for others, although I fully accept that many, many people don't see it that way. Some are out purely to better themselves and their own lives at all costs, whereas others believe this life is just an interview stage to see if they can earn enough points to go on to paradise afterwards. I shall refrain from giving my personal opinion on either of those ways to look at life.

You're welcome.

I know my family would be devastated if I were to lose my life to this cancer, especially in the near future. How do I know? Because I've been through it - with both my Mum and my Dad.

And, to refuse treatment that could delay or even prevent the cancer from striking the fatal blow... that's just being selfish.

My family has to suffer because I'm scared to endure another round of pain, fatigue and utter discomfort? I think I've been brought up to be a better human being than that.

So, listen up universe...

I'll go through anything I have to in order to ensure my family remains happy for as long as possible. I know that, one day, you'll get the upper hand; you will with every one of us. But, until that day comes, the gloves are off, and the fight is on.

See you in the ring.

AND THE REST

O K, now that my treatment is over, I'm going to
take a few days - possibly longer - away from my
computer, this blog, social media and my ongoing,
solid gold membership of Club Penguin, to do... absolutely
nothing.

It's time to slump. It's time to rest. It's time to just be.

I have to forget about work, although the ongoing
inability to write is starting to drive me insane. Writing isn't
just a job; I love it. And I would continue to do it, even if I
wasn't being paid (for many years, that's exactly what I did).
It's like an itch I have to scratch - that also happens to
support my family. (Now all I can think about is becoming a
professional itcher, being paid to ease those little niggles, but
only if my work is up to scratch - WAHEY!)

Imagine if you were a plumber (unless, of course, you are a
plumber - in which case, this will prove to be a very simple
exercise), and someone or something stopped you from
plumbing. Just like it would be if you stopped a singer from
singing, a gardener from gardening, or a dentist from, er...
denting.

I can't wait to get back in the saddle and start writing again (man, my metaphors are getting mixed up today - I'm as confused as a Welsh bowling ball).

Anyhoo - you get my point. I'm signing off for a while to get some much needed rest.

There, why couldn't I just put it that simply to begin with?

Oh, yeah... I'm me.

BARRY - AGAIN!

H ello! Tommy's mate, Barry, here. The more observant among you may have noticed that Tommy hasn't posted much of late. The good news is, he's now finished his treatment   hooray!

The bad news is, it's left him feeling ill. Very ill. So ill, in fact, that he's currently pretty much bed-bound, and unable to get here to blog about his latest experiences himself. Rest assured, though, he'll be back just as soon as he's able.

In the meantime, I thought I'd write a little about another time Tommy was seriously ill, although on this occasion it was as a result of something far less serious than cancer. It was as a result of alcohol. Evil, evil alcohol.

Tommy was living in London at the time, but was up visiting me in the Highlands of Scotland. He was actually appearing in a film I had written and was directing, but that's a story for another time.

After the first day of shooting, we all went out to celebrate at a local pub. There, we had a few very civilised pints, before deciding to try the glittering beverage I offered him.

Goldschlager, in case you don't know, is a sort of

cinnamon liqueur, with lots of little flakes of gold floating around in it. According to some random bloke in the pub, the flecks of gold are designed to lightly slice the back of your throat so that the alcohol reaches your bloodstream faster. Sounds a little dubious to me, but then, if you can't trust random blokes in the pub, who can you trust?

Shortly after our fourth or fifth shot, I turned round to find Tommy had vanished. Just... vanished. Gone. Disappeared without a trace.

I hunted all around the pub for him, checking in the toilets, under tables, and anywhere else I thought he might have ended up. But to no avail.

I broadened the search, stepped outside, then gasped in amazement. The streets were paved with gold! And vomit! Although, not necessarily in that order.

I looked round to find Tommy slumped against the pub wall. He was shimmering from head to toe, and for a moment I thought he was being beamed aboard the Starship Enterprise, but soon realised that, no, he was just covered in Goldschlager-laced vomit, too.

It was decided we'd get a taxi back to mine, where we were all staying. Four of us piled into the taxi, with Tommy propped up against one of the doors in the back. As the taxi trundled the five miles back to my house, Tommy's condition began to deteriorate. Considering his condition at the start of the journey - covered in vomit and semi-conscious - this did not bode well.

Sure enough, about two miles in, Tommy opened the passenger door (while we were travelling at 50mph) so he could puke onto the road. The taxi driver quickly slammed on the brakes, and told us that Tommy couldn't stay in the cab, as the driver didn't want to risk having to get the upholstery dry-cleaned.

And so, at 2am, 3 miles from home in the Highlands of

Scotland, Tommy and I got out of the taxi and alternately walked, staggered and crawled home. I managed to get him up the stairs to bed, and asked if he wanted tea, toast or anything to calm his stomach. He mumbled that no, he didn't, then fell into bed.

I went downstairs, just in time for the house phone to ring. It caught me off guard and I immediately became worried. Who would be phoning my house at 3am? I tentatively picked it up. "Hello?" I said.

"Yeah," said a voice, after a lengthy pause. "I will have some toast."

Fortunately, he bounced back quick and was ready for filming next day. I know you'll all join me in wishing him a speedy recovery on this occasion, too.

NUNS! REVERSE!

I was confused. But not in a way that could be solved by asking for information or looking up facts and figures.

I just didn't know what the hell was happening.

Every time I tried to walk - even just to the bathroom and back - I lost my balance and fell. I recall trying to stop myself during one of these falls by placing a hand on my desk - and missed. As a result, I fell against the corner of the thing, which hit me hard in the side and caused me extra bruising and pain. Due to my throat, I couldn't even call out for help, and was frequently forced to hoist myself up onto my knees and crawl back to my bedroom, where I'd pull myself up using the edge of the bed.

This had been going on for a few days. I'd tried to sit at my desk and write, but every time I tried to type, the result was gobbledegook. Not just bad writing, but utter gibberish.

The same was true of texts I'd been sending to my brother for a few days. Whenever his phone beeped, chances were it would be a message from me along the lines of:

Ver t7t2I]p'.s,kopmrt u8wewr gy38ryhdl;'idd

As I'm not a secret agent working undercover to share state secrets by code - at least not to my knowledge - this was obviously very worrying. Worrying to the point where he would call and leave messages, or text me back and ask what was wrong. Then I would reply with...

M£8y rc2hi y8yt1o cgy4uwgfcjavc becux r73!

Which didn't help much at all, frankly.

My sister was constantly on the 'phone to Kirsty, checking how I was. They both knew that I needed to see a medical professional, and urgently. Thankfully, the district nurse was due at any moment.

She arrived, saw how ill I was and took a blood test, promising to get the doctor out to see me.

While the nurse was taking my blood, my sister called Kirsty again for an update. Then she sent me a text straight after, asking what the district nurse had said to me.

I replied with "What district nurse? I haven't seen a district nurse today!"

Yep, I was that confused. The echo of the nurse's footsteps towards the front door had hardly faded, and I had already forgotten that she'd been.

And then I saw another nurse, standing in the doorway. She came over to where I was sitting and began to check my vitals - pulse, blood pressure, etc.

Except, she wasn't really there.

I was hallucinating.

My imaginary nurse stayed for a while, checking me out, then she left and was replaced by a Nun.

Yep.

The Nun stood in the doorway, praying for me, using her rosary beads.

And no, I have no idea whatsoever why my addled brain conjured up a frighteningly realistic Nun for me to see.

You've probably realised that I'm not a particularly religious person, but I have met and known several Nuns over the course of my life.

My first years at Primary School - then called Infant School - was run and partially staffed by Nuns, as were a lot of similar schools in Liverpool, and around the rest of the UK at that time. The head teacher was a Nun (Sister Something - I wish I could remember her name, although Sister Something sounds like a character from one of my books - so I bagsy it for future use!)

The school was called Park Lane Infants School. I *do* remember that my first teacher was Miss Morley, and that I painted a truck on my first day in her class.

I also remember the one and only time I was taken to see the head teacher because of bad behaviour...

Park Lane Infants School consisted of a real mishmash of buildings. There were red brick classrooms, a two or three story structure where the offices were situated, a row of ramshackle white pebble-dashed classrooms that ran along the side of the playground, and two classrooms that were made of wood, and stood on stilts at one end due to the severe slope in the ground.

One of the most important school rules was that, under no circumstances, were you to go underneath those classrooms. So, of course, kids did exactly that all the time.

Except for me, of course. You see, even at an early age, I was a dedicated, semi-professional coward. The thought of being in trouble with anyone terrifying me to the point of panic attack. I went out of my way to be clearly seen behaving and obeying the rules.

If I went into a shop with my parents or grandparents, I walked around with my hands open, palms up to prove to any suspicious grown-ups that I wasn't there to steal anything (which has just reminded me of another memory - I recall spending pre-decimal currency in those shops! An old penny which, if you don't know, were approximately the side of the Large Hadron Collider, and threepenny bits - the Royal Mint's own ninja throwing stars). So, with all this extreme caution, there was no way I was going to break the rules and go under the cabins, as I think we called them.

Until the day I did.

It was lunchtime, and I was playing with my friends out in the yard. My sister, Sue, had not long started school, and I always tried to spot her and keep an eye on her during break times, like a big brother should. I also made certain to visit the toilet - which was outdoors, and open to the elements! It was essentially just a long wall for the boys to go against. And the entrance/exit was opposite the wooden cabin classrooms...

I remember leaving the toilet and spotting my friend, Paul, peeking out at me from beneath the cabins. It was autumn (I remember because the second, smaller playground which the cabins backed onto, was overlooked by a vast sycamore tree, and we frequently spent our free time catching and throwing the twisting and tumbling sycamore seeds as they fell from the branches.

Sycamore seeds - nature's fidget spinners! (If you're reading this in the distant future, and don't know what a fidget spinner is, imagine a small device that you hold in your hand that spins. That's it. In the age of virtual reality gaming consoles, kids - and adults - are going crazy over colourful bits of metal and plastic and that can spin. Until they stop spinning, and then you can spin them again. It's a wonder the human race ever made it to the Moon...)

Where was I? Oh yes, I'd peed up against a brick wall (simpler times), and spotting my mate, Paul, as I made my way back into the playground. He beckoned me over and urged me to go under the cabin, where he was. I hesitated, my natural fraidy-cat impulses kicking in big time, but then decided 'What the Hell?' You only live once!

So, I threw caution to the wind, and crawled under the wooden classroom.

I'd like to tell you what it was like under there, but I wasn't there long enough for my brain to form a memory. One of the dinner ladies had obviously seen me disappear beneath the structure, and reached under to haul me out, along with Paul and the half dozen other boys currently blowing raspberries to 'the man' and going boldly where no infant was allowed to go.

We were all marched to the head teacher's office, on the second floor of the larger block, and left to wait outside.

Where I instantly began to cry. A lot. I sobbed like a lost baby whose balloon has just burst.

I can even remember my reaction to the other boys (who, somehow, managed not to cry or leak liquid from any other part of their bodies. I was SO glad I'd visited the outside toilet just moments before.) I was the only one crying, so these other kids were clearly hardened criminals, ready to pay their dues to society.

Remember that, back in those days (how old do I sound?) - and this would have been in 1973 or 1974 (strike that, I am old) - corporal punishment was still not only allowed, but encouraged as a way to maintain discipline in schools. Thankfully, the cane was on the wane (like the rain in Spain), but the leather strap was racing up the punishment charts to take its place.

And I knew kids who had been given the strap by Sister Something. On the palm of the hand. Several times. Then, they were sent back to class to try to write with a pencil held in that now red, swollen, aching hand.

Now it was my turn, hence my snot-nosed blubbing.

I clearly recall saying: "She's going to give me the strap, and it's going to hurt!"

No-one replied. So, I carried on crying.

Then, the office door opened, and I lost it. I was in hysterics. I was six years old and, aside from the occasional confrontation at home, I'd never been in trouble before. Now, here I was, starting out on my life of crime and retribution.

We all held out our hands, and Sister Something went down the line...

...giving each of us three jelly babies.

Then she ruffled our hair, told us to be good boys, and sent us back to class.

I don't remember the walk back to my classroom. I think the relief and sheer euphoria that a woman who had devoted her entire life to the church hadn't hit me with a thick lump of leather was simply too much to cope with, and I blanked out the rest of the day.

And I didn't tell my Mum what had happened when she came to pick me and my sister up at home time. I was a genius. I'd got away with it!

Until Sister Something told her about how I'd cried at parents' evening.

Grrr! Nuns!

A few years ago, I was driving through that part of Liverpool with Kirsty and the boys, and I turned down Park Lane to show them the first school I attended. Only it's not there anymore. It's now a housing estate. And, no matter how hard I tried, I couldn't squeeze under any of the houses.

I don't think they liked me peeing up against the wall, either.

That was my first experience with Nuns, and probably the reason why my mind had conjured up a hallucination of one on this occasion.

If you weren't brought up Catholic, you may not be aware that praying through an entire rosary takes ages. So, after a while, I gave up and went upstairs to bed.

And that's when everything went wrong...

VERY DARK

I t was dark.

And not just 'absence of light' dark. It was as though someone had thrown the darkness over me, smothering me in the inability to see. Or even think.

I was aware that there were people nearby. I couldn't tell what they were saying (their voices seemed to be coming from many miles away), but I could tell that they were agitated.

They sounded worried about something.

Then, one of the voices broke through...

"Thomas. Thomas, can you hear me?"

"Yes," I replied.

"Can you open your eyes, Thomas?"

I tried, but couldn't, and told the disembodied voice as much.

"OK," he said. "Do you know where you are right now?"

This one gave me pause to think for a moment. "No," I admitted. "I don't know where I am."

"Thomas, you're in A&E."

I think I actually chuckled then. "No, I'm not!" I said. "Why would I be in A&E?"

And that was it. The voice faded away to mix with the general hubbub and chatter of background noise. The conversation was, apparently, over.

I didn't find out until later, but it was around this time that doctors took Kirsty, my wife, to one side to tell her that the prognosis wasn't good.

After hallucinating both nurses and nuns, I'd gone up to bed at around 4pm, and fell straight to sleep.

I had then, apparently, fallen out of bed in the early hours of the morning and Kirsty had been unable to wake me up. First one, then two ambulance crews were called to carry me downstairs to the gleaming yellow chariot that was to speed me to A&E and then the Intensive Care Unit at Blackburn Hospital.

At that point, the doctors took my family aside and told them that, unless I started responding very soon, I had approximately two hours left to live.

Two hours. I'm so glad I didn't know that.

My blood pressure had plummeted to dangerously low levels. The oxygen in my bloodstream was at 35%. I was seriously ill, and unconscious.

I was dying.

The doctors considered putting me into a medically induced coma and ventilating me - hesitating only because they were uncertain that I would ever come out of it.

Eventually, after giving me regular small doses of medication to try to raise my blood pressure, I began to stabilise and the threat to life reduced to the point where I could be left in the care of ICU nurses.

Not that I knew anything about this.

I regained consciousness several hours later, and found myself in an unfamiliar bed, linked up to any number of drips, monitors and other flashing, beeping machines and other sci-fi looking paraphernalia.

For some reason, I believed I was in a factory, overseeing the production of golden robots.

Hey, they're my hallucinations! And robots are better than nuns.

Unless they're robot nuns.

I became aware of someone else in the room. It was a nurse. A real one! She helped me to have a sip of water, and told me where I was. It wasn't until later in the day that I was told why I was here...

I had double pneumonia and sepsis. And it had almost killed me.

Kirsty arrived back at the hospital that afternoon, having had to nip home to see to our sons, Arran and Sam. I called her closer and half-croaked, half-whispered to her...

"I think I'm in the intensive care unit."

"Yes," she said, her eyes flooding with tears. "Yes, you are."

"And, I think I might be very ill this time..."

I can still feel the hug she gave me.

For a long time, I found it very difficult to stop thinking about what might have happened if Kirsty hadn't heard me fall out of bed.

BARRY'S BACK!

Hello all.

I'm sure you're all keen to hear the latest on Tommy's condition.

Thirty-six hours ago, Tommy's blood oxygen was critically low, and doctors were preparing to induce coma and place him on a ventilator. However, Tommy came out of his corner swinging, and during that night his blood oxygen levels began to rise.

Yesterday, he opened his eyes and sat up, and was able to interact with his family and the hospital staff. After a bit of a coughing fit, his voice even returned for a few seconds, and he was able to very briefly speak to his brother, Bryan, who was with him at the time.

Tommy's sister, Sue, had been keeping me updated via text message throughout the day, and when she told me that Tommy now had his phone with him, I decided to fire off a message of my own, just letting him know I was thinking of him. An hour or so later, my phone bleeped.

You think an aggressive cancer, six weeks of gruelling

treatment, an infection and pneumonia in both lungs is going to keep Tommy Donbavand down? Nah!

While everyone is hugely relieved at the improvement he has shown, doctors have warned that he's not out of the woods yet, and there's a long road to recovery ahead. He's still in the critical unit, isolated in his own room. As well as the pneumonia, his burns have become infected, and his immune system is in no condition to battle either of those things. He could take a turn for the worse at any time, but right now he's awake, he's (mostly) alert, and he's alive.

Or so they tell him, at least.

I SEE YOU, ICU

In total, I spent a week in the intensive care unit at Blackburn Hospital.

I was in a room by myself, strapped up to all manner of beeping and flashing machines, and with a weird tentacle like contraption in the corner. I later found out that this was a portable winch, that the staff had on standby in case they couldn't manually lift me into bed. (I was still considerably overweight at this stage).

There was also a respirator, that would have helped me to breathe if the doctors had followed through with their plan to put me into a medically induced coma. They eventually decided against that option, as the chances were good that I wouldn't come out of it, and I would spend the rest of what little life I had left in that vegetative state.

Thankfully, the horrifically low oxygen levels in my blood eventually rallied to a point where the coma became unnecessary.

I was diagnosed with double pneumonia and sepsis.

I'd had pneumonia several times before, and had been

hospitalised because of it four times previously. However, I'd never had it this badly, nor in both lungs at the same time.

I didn't know what sepsis was, but a quick search of Wikipedia told me what I needed to know...

Sepsis is a life-threatening condition that arises when the body's response to infection causes injury to its own tissues and organs. Common signs and symptoms include fever, increased heart rate, increased breathing rate, and confusion.

Sound familiar?

The question was, how had I managed to pick this up? The cause was most likely the nasty burn mark the radiotherapy sessions had left all around my neck. It had become infected and, coupled with my now virtually non-existent immune system (thanks again, radiotherapy), it spread throughout my body like wildfire.

It was several days before I was able to come off the oxygen feed and breathe satisfactorily on my own. I was producing lots of mucus, that threatened to choke me, so I had a suction tube to help with that. I'd been fitted with a catheter to take care of those issues, and I was connected to a feed pump to ensure I received the correct nutrients via my peg tube.

Kirsty, Sue (my sister), Bryan (my brother) and several aunts and uncles popped in to visit me, but I was unable to conduct any real conversations with them, so I mainly just lay in bed and listened to them chat among themselves.

On one occasion, Kirsty brought Arran and Sam in to visit me. I was amazed at how well they coped with seeing me in that condition. Unfortunately, that was soon to change as Sam in particular began to worry excessively about my state of health. More on that in another post, coming soon.

When I could croak out a few words, I asked Kirsty for more details about what had happened to me. From my point of view, I had been at home, seeing imaginary nuns, and then nothing but a few lines of conversation while the doctors tried to resuscitate me, until I eventually came to in what I believed was a factory making golden robots.

What she told me was, if anything, even more insane...

As I mentioned previously, the district nurse had come out to see me, and had taken a blood sample. She agreed with both Kirsty and Sue that I needed to see a doctor as a matter of urgency, so she called the surgery I was registered with, and left a message to ask the duty doctor to pay me a visit.

She didn't hear anything back.

So, she called again, later that afternoon. Once again, she called the surgery and repeated her request for the duty doctor to come out to me.

Once again - silence.

So, at the end of her shift, she drove to the surgery, went inside and told the doctor face to face it was very important that he visit me.

But, he didn't do that.

Instead, he made an appointment for a different doctor at the surgery - my now friend, Dr Ellison, to visit me the following lunchtime.

Before which time, I almost died.

Yep, that's right.

I almost died because the duty doctor couldn't be arsed to come out and see me as the nurse had insisted. If he *had* come out, he would no doubt have been able to spot the tell-tale signs of sepsis, and arranged for an ambulance.

But, he didn't.

I should mention here that I do know the name of the doctor who very nearly saw me off, but I won't mention it. Legal action may still be an option.

Once Dr Ellison discovered what had happened - that the duty doctor had decided I wasn't worth the trip and what had happened as a result, she resigned from the surgery. She later told me it was the last in a long line of problems she'd had to deal with while working there. My situation was the last straw.

So, there you have it. The reason I came within two hours of death.

And that reason was a doctor.

VERY LIGHT

I've been thinking hard about my recent update – the one about being surrounded by darkness and hearing distant voices while I was unconscious in the resuscitation room at Blackburn Hospital.

I read through the post again and again, but something didn't sit right with me. Something felt wrong, but I couldn't put my finger on what it was.

So, I closed my eyes, and ran through what little I could remember of that night.

Then it hit home. I realised what I was getting wrong.

And that realisation knocked the wind out of me.

It was the darkness I mentioned. You see, it wasn't dark at all.

It was light.

Bright white light.

Holy crap!

I'd been heading for the light when the doctor's voice broke through to me.

I remember beginning to die.

Thinking about that while being aware that the medical

staff told my family that I had around two hours left to live unless I started to respond quickly, and it all adds up.

That was it.

That was the tunnel of light many people claim to have seen during near death experiences.

The tunnel of bright, white light.

Now, I'm not saying that's an entrance to Heaven, or the face of God himself, or anything like that. I'm not a religious person and, as such, I don't expect there to be an afterlife (unless it transpires that we're all exhibits in a vast alien zoo or future human computer simulation).

Perhaps it's the brain firing off bursts of electrical impulses in an effort to shock itself back into life like some dense, neural defibrillator, or the connections from the eyes zapping signals back and forth in a moment of crisis.

Who knows?

Whatever it is, I experienced it - and my consciousness tried valiantly to hide it from me. But, I could just feel that something was out of place with my recollection of that night.

Knowing how close I came to leaving this world - and my family - behind isn't a pleasant memory to have, and part of me wishes it had stayed buried. However, I've decided to use it as a warning; a reminder to ask for help the next time I feel that something is wrong, rather than try to muddle through.

It's obvious that I was in a far worse state than I had originally believed. And that's a situation I can't allow to happen again.

WARD 1

After a week in intensive care, I was considered well enough to be transferred up to a normal ward. And so, I was.

I can't remember the name of the ward, but it was one of the larger men's wards - and one I'd stayed in on at least two occasions previously. Both times while suffering from pneumonia.

I was one of twelve men on the ward, and was given a bed halfway along one side, under a window. By now, we were well into what was proving to be a glorious summer - not that I knew a lot about it, having spent most of the good weather in hospital.

One of the problems with being in hospital is visiting. Although I only live around 13 miles from Blackburn Hospital, that's 13 miles across country, and it's not an easy journey to make unless by car.

Kirsty doesn't drive.

The obvious solution would be to travel by public transport, but that would require two bus journeys totalling anything up to two and a half hours - each way. Plus, there would be a considerable walk from our home to the stop where the first bus can be caught.

I wasn't keen on her doing that, for obvious reasons, especially as she would be making the journey alone. Plus, she had two kids to look after full time as I wasn't around to help.

So, it came down to taxis. And that wasn't easy, either. Using taxis proved to be very expensive - £25 ($33) in each direction. Even if Kirsty only came to see me during one of the two visiting sessions each day, it would still cost £50 ($65) for the round trip, or £350 ($450) per week.

That's a lot of money, especially when you consider that I was (and still am) the only wage earner in our household, and the pause button had been pressed on that particular activity.

Friends and family rallied around to help whenever they could, and I remain eternally grateful to each and every one of them for their kindness and generosity in picking up Kirsty, and bringing her to visit me for an hour or two.

If you've ever stayed in hospital, you'll know just how lonely and depressing it can be. You're ill and feeling low to begin with, but add being away from home and missing family on top of that, and it's not a good mix.

To make things worse, I was so drained by what I'd just been through, that I would await Kirsty's arrival with excitement, then fall asleep once she arrived. After a few days, she began to bring a book along with her so that, if I did doze off, she could sit with me and read.

The first week of my stay on the ward was relatively unremarkable, although the pneumonia resulted in my having to use a nebuliser regularly (a gadget that pumps a mixture of air, saline water and occasionally asthma medication to a face mask). Most of the time, I was simply bored. I read as much as I could take, occasionally watched a Euro 2016 football match on the bedside TV system, and started to watch catch up TV on the BBC iPlayer with my iPad.

Which had quite a weird effect...

THE SIZE OF IT

One of the side effects of the cancer and resulting treatment is that I've been unable to eat properly for quite some time. In fact, the last time I had a meal by mouth was on 1st May.

All I've had to eat since then are NHS milkshakes via my stomach peg.

I'm SO fed up with milkshakes!

They come in an assortment of flavours (not that I can taste them), and eat provide essential vitamins and nutrients plus 300 calories of energy.

Yummy!

That's not to say I haven't tried eating normally. I underwent a swallow test at the hospital a few weeks ago and given the go ahead to start eating solids again - but it's just too painful.

I've tried thin soups, bouillon, Bovril and watery chicken and vegetable stock.

Too painful.

I've tried baby food, runny eggs and finely cut up pieces of meat.

Too painful.

And so, I'm still on these blasted milkshakes!

And the worst part about it?

I'M SO HUNGRY!

The food Kirsty makes for herself and the boys smells so utterly delicious, and on the odd occasion when they've ordered a takeaway to be delivered...

AARRRGGGHH!

As it is, I'm now looking forward to a Christmas dinner that Kirsty will blend in the NutriBullet so I can pour it down my stomach tube. Liquid turkey, potatoes, sprouts and parsnips.

And I REALLY miss cheese!

SIGH!

Still, there has been one positive result from sticking to such a strict liquid diet for so long - the weight loss.

When I was first diagnosed with cancer, I was at my all-time heaviest. I've been overweight for much of my adult life but, at the start of this year, it had reached the stage where my weight was out of control and very dangerous.

I never used to admit this to anyone, as I was ashamed to do so. But, I weighed in at 22 stone 4 pounds (141kg or 312 pounds).

Disgusting!

And I felt it. Day to day activities were difficult, I was out of breath all the time, I suffered from sleep apnoea, and I looked a mess in my 4XL or even 5XL shirts and 56 inch trousers.

Then I found out I had cancer, which probably saved my life.

As of today, I weigh 11 stone 1 pound.

I've lost just over 11 stones - or half my entire body weight.

I've had to buy new clothes. My shirts are now XL or 2XL (depending on the make), and I'm in 38 inch trousers.

And - aside from all the cancer stuff - I feel great!

Of course, losing so much weight in such a short period of time is not recommended by any medical professional. And I wouldn't suggest 'The Cancer Plan' as a diet routine for anyone.

But it has, quite possibly, saved me from an early death.

Talk about irony...

WARD 2

During my second week on the main ward, I started to feel very depressed. I was missing Kirsty and the boys dreadfully, and even though I got to see Kirsty almost every day, there were days when we there wasn't anyone available to give her a lift, and we couldn't afford to spend yet another £50 on the taxi journey. When that happened, I sat beside my hospital bed alone while everyone else welcomed their family and friends.

On the second day of week two, a new patient was moved into the bed opposite me. He was seriously unwell. In addition to whichever nasty ailment had caused his hospital stay, he suffered with a terrible skin condition that caused it to blister, peel and hurt to the point where he couldn't get out of bed, or walk.

The doctors were planning to send him to a care home to recuperate in the long term, and this clearly upset him. He alternated between snapping at any of the nurses who tried to help him, frequently resorting to racist insults, and calling home to sob for hours at a time to his wife. He was in a bad way and, while I sympathised with his situation, I didn't like the way he spoke to the nurses – who were universally wonderful – and the constant crying did nothing to help my own depression.

I feel very selfish about writing that, but it's true. I was ill and down and sadly, this guy's attitude wasn't helping me. Quite the opposite, in fact.

So, I immersed myself in watching TV shows on my iPad. Through the BBC iPlayer app, I started to watch the series *Death in Paradise* from the very beginning. For those who don't know, *Death in Paradise* follows the cases of a British murder detective who is transferred to run the tiny police force on the fictional Caribbean island of Saint Marie. The show originally starred Ben Miller, then Kris Marshall and, presently, Ardal O'Hanlon.

I watched episodes back to back (thankfully, there were plenty of them), most of the time wearing my headphones to drown out the ruckus from across the way. As I was feeding with milkshakes via my peg tube, I didn't even have to stop for meal breaks (although I started to become very envious whenever the food trolley made an appearance!)

I was having blood test after blood test (or, at least, that's what it felt like) and, after a while, I didn't even stop my viewing for those. I just held out my arm whenever a phlebotomist approached my bed.

I should add a short side note here... I have terrible veins. They're thin, deep below the surface, and hard to find. VERY hard to find. For my entire stay in hospital, the chances of staff getting blood on their first attempt happened maybe half a dozen times. On every other occasion, it took two, three or even more attempts to find a working vein. This was another reason why I took to watching *Death in Paradise* while they closed their eyes and stabbed needles in my arms.

On several occasions, they were forced to resort to taking blood from the back of my hands, or from my feet. If you've never experienced that, let me tell you that both of those options really sodding hurts! By now, my body was covered with blossoming black and purple bruises.

You may recall that I had been warned not to play my favourite music to help me through my many radiotherapy sessions - the reason being that I would begin to associate the music with the treatment, making it impossible for me to listen to it any longer.

I will admit that I was sceptical. I'm relatively smart, I can distance my personal likes and dislikes from whatever experience I'm going through.

But, it's true.

I don't watch a lot of TV, but I enjoy police procedural dramas, especially those with an unusual premise like *Death in Paradise*. However, the more I watched of the series, the more I began to feel uneasy every time the opening credits began to roll. All I could think about was the sensation of being weak, fatigued and ill. My neck and throat would begin to throb, and I'd feel short of breath. And I could imagine the 'sharp scratch' on my arm as a member of staff attempted to locate one of my veins and collect a blood sample.

All because of a TV show.

In the end, I had to stop watching *Death in Paradise*, and even writing about it now is making me feel anxious.

I'm so glad I didn't decide to watch *Doctor Who* while I was there!

And then I was told I was being discharged. This came as a surprise as I certainly didn't feel as though I was well enough to go home. I told the doctors and nurses how I felt, but the decision had been made. Recovered or not, I was heading back to Kirsty and the boys. This made me happy, but also extremely concerned in case I suffered another set-back and ended up back in hospital.

Little did I know...

SMACK DOWN

Kirsty arrived in a taxi to pick me up from hospital. I'd already packed my bags and received the medication I was due to leave with, so it wasn't long before we were on our way.

She took me down to the taxi in a wheelchair, as I was still unable to walk any further than the bathroom and back - and even that was a struggle. And, less than an hour later, I was back at home.

It was so wonderful to see Arran and Sam again. I'd missed them both so much. I'd called them frequently from my hospital bed - normally though a FaceTime video call where they would tell me what they'd been up to at school and college, or show me their work and whatever they'd been doing at home.

As I've already mentioned, I didn't feel well enough to come home, but I was determined to get plenty of rest now that I was. So, after being back for just 20 minutes, I decided to go up to bed for a nap.

This brought back a lot of strange feelings. The last time I'd slept in my own bed, I'd fallen out and Kirsty hadn't been able to rouse me. So, it was with a feeling of nervousness that I made for the stairs.

Kirsty told me to wait so she could help me up to bed. But, I figured, I had to learn how to do this again. I couldn't rely on someone helping me around the house for the rest of my life. Besides, I had the bannisters to hold. What could possibly go wrong?

The answer is - a lot.

A lot could go wrong, and it did.

I got as far as the second step, and then I fell. Backwards. Onto the hard hall floor. Pain shot through my body and took my breath away.

Kirsty tried to help me sit up, but every movement was agony; whatever I had done was causing lightning bolts to shoot up and down my back.

Eventually, I managed to flip myself over and I crawled into the living room where I used the arm of the sofa to pull myself upright. I slumped down and asked Kirsty to get me some painkillers. I'd been an idiot.

Over the next couple of hours, I began to find it harder and harder to breathe until, eventually, Kirsty called another ambulance.

A motorbike paramedic arrived first. He checked me out and discovered that the oxygen levels in my blood had plummeted yet again. He called through to make sure the ambulance was on its way.

That arrived a few minutes later - and then I was whisked back to hospital. I was taken back into the resuscitation room in A&E, the very place where I'd been unconscious three weeks earlier and, through my croaks and wheezes, tried to explain that I'd only been discharged a few hours earlier.

I was taken for an x-ray which showed I had managed to fracture a rib in my fall. How lucky am I?!

I was moved to the medical assessment unit for further tests and, eventually, up to a different, smaller ward. This room only had six beds, and I was in the far, right corner.

By now, it was the early hours of the morning. The other patients were all asleep, so the nurse in charge had to attempt to take a blood sample - from my virtually non-existent veins - by the light of a single lamp above my bed. It took five or six attempts but she got there in the end and left to drop the blood samples off to go to the lab.

But, in the dark, she hadn't secured the cap on the end of my cannula (the little tube they insert into your vein for each access when attaching you to a drip, etc.) properly. It popped off, disappearing into the darkness somewhere, and the cannula started to stray a tall plume of my blood high into the air.

I'll admit that I panicked, attempting to stem the flow while calling for someone to help me while not waking any of my fellow patients. Some welcome to the ward they'd give me if I turned up shouting and pissing blood all over them.

It took a while but, eventually, someone heard my cries for help, and the situation was rectified. I then changed out of my blood-soaked pyjamas, feeling glad this hadn't happened just before visiting time, and finally settled down to try to get some sleep.

I was back in hospital, and my state of mind was only going to keep on deteriorating before it got any better.

WARD 3

I settled in to the new ward relatively quickly. It was a lot quieter than the previous ward, partly down to the fact that there were only six beds, but also because two of my fellow patients slept virtually all the time, and the others either listened to the radio or TV with headphones, or read books.

To amuse myself, I began to give the other patients names and identities, just to amuse myself. I've spent years either playing other characters on stage, or inventing them for my books – so this kind of stuff pops into my head quite frequently, and often without warning.

Please understand, however, that I'm not in any way trying to ridicule these individuals, or be mean about them. I was simply very bored, and invented fictional details about them as a way to pass the time.

So, going around the ward in order, I'd like to introduce you to...

In bed one, we have one of our sleepers – at least for the first few days. Then he was replaced with Dougie, who I'll get to later.

In bed two, there was Clifford, The Big Red Pensioner. Cliff was an elderly gent who also slept a lot, but had the largest face and bald head combination I've ever seen. He looked like he was a giant light bulb from the neck up - and his face was such a violent shade of red that he virtually glowed in the dark. When he was sleeping, he also had a tendency to slide down in his bed, until only the large, red dome of his cranium was visible. At that point, he became one of Roger Hargreaves' abandoned early concept drawings of *The Mr Men*.

For those that don't know, *The Mr Men* is a series of wonderful children's books created by the late Roger Hargreaves and now continued by his son, Adam, along with their female equivalents in *The Little Miss* series. They included such now classic characters as *Mr Bump*, *Mr Happy* and *Little Miss Chatterbox*.

Most recently, the format has been extended to include versions of the titular Time Lord in my favourite TV show, *Doctor Who*. Currently published are *Doctor First*, *Doctor Fourth*, *Doctor Eleventh* and *Doctor Twelfth*, with more on the way!

If you've never come across *The Mr Men* series before, I highly recommend searching for them online and picking up a copy or two for the young children in your life. I guarantee they will love them as much as I did, and as did both of my sons, Arran and Sam.

Many years ago, when I was in *Buddy: The Buddy Holly Story* in London, I lived in a flat on the edge of Pimlico, just behind Victoria Coach Station. One of my neighbours (whose name I can't recall) was the narrator of *The Mr Men* audio books, having taken over from the late, great Arthur Lowe.

Anyhoo - back to my hospital ward...

Next to Cliff was the gent I shall refer to as 'A Child's Drawing of Ricky Gervais', as that's exactly what he resembled. It was as though this poor guy had the misfortune to be born without a face - just an empty expanse of skin. In an effort to help the poor guy to fit into society, a passing four year old had helpfully pulled out his set of crayons, and attempted to rectify the situation by quickly sketching the best rendition he could of writer and comedian, Ricky Gervais. The result was poor, to say the least. And wasn't helped by this patient's utter refusal to allow the nurses to help him do anything - from cutting up his food, to using the frame they had provided to get to and from the bathroom. As a result, virtually everything he attempted failed spectacularly with slapstick level results.

Switching over to the other side of the ward, there was me (who you've already met) and, next door, Beardy Crisp Man.

Beardy Crisp Man listened to the radio a lot, and he had a trim beard. Which seemed to be about all there was to him - until, on my second night in the ward, his son arrived for a visit at just after midnight - long after the official visiting hours had ended.

This appeared to have been pre-arranged with the nurses as it was clear this was the only time he could get to the hospital to see his Dad, and the visits continued night after night. However, they were fleeting get-togethers, lasting only five or ten minutes, and the purpose of which appeared to be to hand over two or three packets of crisps, ask after each other's well-being, and then it was time to get out of there.

Night after night, the son would show up, say hello to the nurses, hand his father a few packets of crisps - sometimes ready salted, other times cheese and onion flavoured and, on one rather extremely memorable occasion, a selection of Wotsits - say 'How are you?', then it was all over. While I was there, they didn't discuss anything other than the type of crisps wanted on the next visit.

The final patient in the ward slept for the entire time I was there, so I nicknamed him Reginald. Although his real name was Steven. I don't know either.

All in all, it was a very peaceful set up - until the first sleeper mentioned was moved to a different ward, and we got Dougie.

Bloody hell. Dougie.

Dougie had... problems. A lot of problems. He was an extremely short Glaswegian chap (not that either of those are problems, as such), with a temper that could rival Mount Vesuvius on eruption day.

He'd fallen at home and broken his hip and, as such, he was restricted to bed. But that's not what Dougie wanted. Dougie wanted to be up and about, even though he couldn't walk due to his injury. But that didn't stop him from trying to get up at least twice per minute, then complaining loudly and profanely at the top of his voice when each and every attempt at leaving his bed failed.

He yelled at the other patients, the nurses, the doctors, the visitors, the chairs, the windows, the sheets, the curtains, the nitrogen atoms in the air, and anything else he believed he could or could not see.

All day. Every day.

It got to the stage where an extra member of staff was hired to sit at his bedside 24 hours a day to try to stop him from getting up. This always ended up in a cartoon fist fight - like those you see in comics that consist simply of a cloud with hands and feet protruding from it at weird angles.

And these poor sods who were employed especially to keep Dougie from breaking his other hip were almost all doctor or nursing students, trying to earn an extra bit of income to help pay their way through medical school. I know this because they all brought text books and notepads along with them to get some work done while sitting at their allotted patient's bedside, not that they ever got to open any of them.

After two or three days of Dougie's constant antics (he never seemed to sleep, so why should the rest of us?), myself and Beardy Crisp Man could take it no longer and appealed to the nurses for help. Both Reginald and Clifford, The Big Red Pensioner could have slept through an earthquake, and A Child's Drawing of Ricky Gervais refused to join our mini-revolution, as that would mean admitting to the staff that he needed help, and he absolutely, certainly didn't.

BCM and I remained calm, and explained to the ward sister that, while we empathised with Dougie's unhappiness with his situation, we weren't getting any of the rest or sleep that was vital to our own recoveries. She agreed, and so from that night, Dougie and whichever unfortunate student turned up to be his unwilling sparring partner (none of them ever came back a second time), were moved out into a corridor at lights out. You could still hear his ranting, echoing off in the distance, but it was finally possible to sleep through it.

A few days later, I managed to pick up a stomach bug - and that meant I had to be moved to another ward so that I wouldn't inadvertently pass on my infection to any of my other chums.

And so, I waved this part of my adventure a fond goodbye.

WARD 4

This time, I was moved to one of the more modern wards in the hospital - and given a room of my own! With a bathroom of my own! That was the best part, I have to admit. No more wading through pungent pools of pensioner piss several times a day. That had to be a good thing.

And it was a good thing. At first.

Then, after a day or two, I began to feel exceptionally lonely.

I love a bit of peace and quiet as much as the next cancer sufferer who is visited by hallucinatory nuns and was only saved from certain death by falling out of bed in the early hours of the morning. But this was too much.

What made it worse was that this ward was positioned in a part of the hospital that wasn't covered by the public wi-fi.

Yes, in case you didn't know, the NHS now provides free wi-fi for its patients and their visitors. You just have to log in, and then you can happily post as many selfies in oxygen masks as your little heart desires.

I'd been using the wi-fi not only to keep in touch with

family and friends, and to watch movies and TV as a way to pass the time (see my previous post about my experience with the BBC detective series, *Death in Paradise*), but also to make and receive video calls to Kirsty, Arran and Sam. While I could do that, I didn't feel too bad. I missed them, of course, but at least we were in touch on a daily basis. Now, that simply wasn't possible. Not even through my phone's 3G access, which was about as useful as a lifeboat on a teapot.

And, no matter how much of a technophile I am, even I wouldn't stoop to the level of asking to be moved to a ward with better wi-fi access.

Kirsty came up with a plan, whereby she would take my iPad home every other night after she visited, and download a handful of movies for me to watch when she returned with it the next day. Then, the day after, she'd take it home again and repeat the process. It wasn't perfect, but it helped.

So, I started to read more to pass the time, and quickly got through many of the books I had with me. Then, one day, the nurse popped in to say I had a visitor. This was in the morning, way before the scheduled visiting hours, so she asked me to go with her down to an unused day room to meet with whoever had come to see me - so that the other patients wouldn't see visitors passing their doorways and want to know why they couldn't have people in to see them 'out of hours'.

At this stage, I didn't know who had come to see me. So, the nurse helped me along the corridor to see my cousin Mark and his son, Josh! They'd driven all the way from Liverpool to see me, unaware that this ward had specific and quite strictly kept visiting hours (each ward at Blackburn Hospital was allowed to arrange and manage their own individual visiting schedules). The distance travelled was the reason the nurse hadn't simply turned them away.

I hadn't seen either of them in months, so it was great to

chat (even with my barely understandable voice) and catch up.

Plus, Mark had brought a handful of books in for me! What a fella!

As I've previously mentioned on many occasions, I'd been unable to eat for several months and was still pouring those bloody milkshakes down my stomach tube to survive. In hospital terms, this is known as 'Nil By Mouth', and a sign to indicate as such was posted prominently over each of my several beds.

One of the few advantages to being in a private room was that I didn't have to sit, watch and endure the smell while the staff dished out meals for the other patients. Meals which, perhaps not the most appetising in the world (hospital food does have something of a poor reputation, after all), was still better than those poxy milkshakes!

When you are able to eat the food, one of the nurses hands out a menu and a pencil each afternoon. This lists the food choices for the following day, and patients are instructed to mark off their choices for breakfast, lunch and dinner. If you're unlucky enough to have just taken possession of a bed after another patient has been discharged, you are generally obliged to contend with whatever they had chosen, thinking they would still be there to enjoy it. But that was only for the first day of your stay and, if you know you're about to be heading home, you can have a bit of naughty fun by choosing some weird combination of foodstuffs to be served to whoever takes your place. Curried peaches, anyone?

As a milkshake user, this wasn't something I had to deal with during my initial month's stay. But, for whatever reason, the nurse who had the task of handing out the daily menus on this ward brought one to my room *every single day*.

I spoke to her, politely explaining that I didn't need such a thing (I didn't want to hurt her feelings by saying that I really didn't want a daily reminder of what I couldn't eat three times a day, after all), to which she simply smiled and said, "Just choose whatever you would have liked to have eaten, and imagine that while you're having your milkshakes!"

It's amazing how deep you can push a pencil into another person's eyeball, isn't it?

Disclaimer: I did not really attempt to blind a nurse by attacking her with an item of stationery.

All in all, I spent a week in my single room and then, finally, I was discharged and allowed to go home.

Aside from less than half a day back at home (which I only visited so I could take a dive down the stairs and fracture a rib), I had now been in hospital for just over a month. I was really ready to leave.

And I did. For a few days, at least.

LIVING IT UP, DOWNSTAIRS

Finally, I was at home. I was so glad to be back with Kirsty and the boys. This time, I was encouraged by the district nurses to sleep downstairs in an effort to avoid any further accidents.

This I did by settling down into an armchair, and resting my legs on a large footstool, which turned out to be a very comfortable set-up. I frequently felt lonely again after everyone said goodnight and vanished upstairs to sleep, leaving me alone, but it was comforting to know that they my family were all under the same roof as me. And, even if I couldn't sleep, I now had access to wi-fi again, so I could spend the wee hours watching movies if I wanted to.

I still couldn't eat or drink, and was still feeding myself by pouring bottles of nutrient-rich milkshakes down my stomach peg. I'd learned to be cautious when doing this, and tried to spread out my feeding sessions as too much liquid in one go was starting to make me feel - and sometimes, be - sick. My wonderful nutritionist at the hospital, Cara, wanted me to get up to six milkshakes a day, at the bare minimum. But that was simply too much.

I was able to handle between two and four bottles a day if I didn't want to risk bringing the stuff straight back up again. And let me tell you, while the flavour of the milkshakes had little to no effect on me while pouring them down the tube into my stomach, it made all the difference when they were coming back in the opposite direction, via the more traditional route. Then, I could really taste the difference between the chocolate and banana varieties.

Which was another thing. I think I may have already mentioned that I don't have a sweet tooth, and never have. Yet, the only flavours of milkshakes available to me were along the lines of strawberry, vanilla, banana and chocolate. There was a companion line in nutritional juices, but they were hard to come by and were still sweet tasting flavours like Apple and Blackcurrant.

During this time, the provider of these meal replacement drinks to the NHS was changed, and the new company offered vanilla, tropical fruit and cappuccino flavours to the mix. Finally, a milkshake that didn't taste like an explosion in a sugar factory!

Once again, I didn't really get to experience the flavour aspect of my 'meals' unless I burped, or worse. Then the tastes hit me hard. What I would have done for a protein packed soup option to be available. Chicken, tomato, beef! But, I could only dream.

Still – no complaining! I was finally home, sleeping comfortably downstairs, using the downstairs bathroom for my ablutions, and now – at last – able to get some rest and get better.

And then I started coughing up blood.

COUGH IT UP

I'd been coughing up blood for a few days when I finally got to see my cancer specialist. The district nurses - and a special, possibly militarised wing of the organisation in darker blue uniforms - had visiting me once or twice a day to make sure I was coping. And, my doctor friend, Dr Ellison, now at her new position in a surgery several miles away, kept a regular eye on me.

I seemed to be OK, but the blood I was producing was a worry. Thankfully, I had an appointment scheduled with Mr Morar (a level above Dr Biswas) in a few days' time.

I've always found it unusual that those who set out on the amazing career path of looking after other people's health train for years and years to finally achieve the status of 'doctor'. Then some of them continue with their training to specialist consultant level where they are allowed to drop the term 'doctor', and become Mr, Mrs or Ms, once again. Surely there needs to be title above doctor that would be appropriate. Overclinician, Uberdoctor, or Supermakerbetterer, perhaps?

No? Ah, well...

So, I had an appointment scheduled with Ultradoctor Morar and told him about the fact that I was coughing up blood. He decided to find out more, and took me into a room which I've never liked going into, ever since this whole nasty business first started.

In this room is a trolley which holds a large monitor screen, and attached to that monitor is a camera through which Mr Morar can examine my throat from the inside. But, it's not like the camera that was used when I had my stomach peg fitted. Oh no. This one doesn't go in via the mouth... (I'll stop you there, just in case you are genuinely concerned that a trained professional is about to stick a length of fiberoptic cable up my arse to examine my throat. It's not that.)

No, this camera goes up my nose, and then down my throat. It's one of the most uncomfortable things I have ever experienced, and Mr Morar loves the bloody thing. He uses it at every sodding opportunity. However, this time, I was genuinely concerned about the blood I was coughing up, so I decided to grit my teeth (which I could do, because the camera went in via my nostril) and bear it.

The result wasn't good. The blood appeared to be coming from one of my lungs. Mr Morar admitted me back into hospital there and then.

WARD 5

I was back inside!

And back in a single room, on the ward next to the ward I had only left a few days earlier. Was this nightmare never going to end?

What followed was day after day of more blood tests, chest x-rays and scans, including a bronchoscopy - where a camera is passed down my throat and directly into my lungs.

Now, I've had many types of hospital scans over the years, especially since first being diagnosed. But the idea of a camera going into my lungs absolutely terrified me.

When the time for me to have the scan arrived, I was taken to a different ward for the day. The ward sister could obviously tell that I was scared, because at one point, she stopped everyone bustling around and preparing me so she could give me a big hug. That made me feel a little letter.

The scan itself was strange and uncomfortable, but not as bad as I had expected. I was helped to sit completely upright, then propped up with boards. I tilted my head back as far as it would go, then the camera was lowered into my mouth and down my throat. Thankfully, there are no nerve endings inside the lungs, so I wasn't actually able to feel the camera diving in and out of my individual bronchial tubes.

One thing I had explained to the scanning team that I didn't want was to see the monitor during the scan. While I'm certain some patients may find it absolutely fascinating to watch the exploration of the insides of their own bodies, I can't think of anything worse. What if it turned out there was a problem, and I was able to see it myself, live on TV? I know I wouldn't be able to cope.

Unfortunately, like many of the scans I've had over the years, the operator of the camera (plus the DP, sound guy, focus puller, key grip and lighting crew) tend to stand near the opening they are using as an entrance for their work, and the monitor is angled towards them. This usually means it's also right in front of me. Thankfully, ever since getting a glimpse of my interior pipework during my first ever colonoscopy, I've learned to keep my eyes tight shut while the procedure is underway. I also keep my fingers crossed that no-one on the medical team feels the need to cry out, "Jesus Christ! What the hell is that?!" or similar exclamations should anything be amiss.

After the bronchoscopy, I was wheeled into the recovery room to sleep off the sedative and throat numbing agent I'd been given for a few hours. This reminds me of the first time I ever had a gastroscopy (camera down my throat and into my stomach). Again, I was very nervous in the run up to the event itself, although one of the nurses was kind enough to explain that she would be coating my throat with 15 sprays of a strong, numbing anaesthetic spray, and that I wouldn't feel the camera (which, by the way, is as thick as a piece of rope) sliding down my throat.

That really helped to settle my nerves until, after the third of the 15 sprays, someone reading my notes said, "Stop!

He's asthmatic!" and everybody very suddenly looked worried.

It transpired that their particular anaesthetic spray of choice wasn't to be used on patients with asthma. Those patients were to be rendered unconscious. But now, that was too late and - despite only having one fifth of the numbness I should have been given - they went ahead with the procedure anyway.

I. Felt. Everything.

It was horrible, and is possibly the reason why I've been so nervous about all subsequent events I've had to attend that end with the suffix -oscopy.

You'll be pleased to learn that the results of the test were clear. But possibly not so pleased when you realise that means the doctors still didn't know why I was coughing up blood.

More scans were needed. So, I stayed in hospital.

One good thing that happened while I was on this ward was a surprise visit from Paul Mills, a friend and my former director from my days in *Buddy*. He was in the north west, directing a show in Warrington, and drove over to surprise me during an afternoon off. It was so wonderful to see him. We'd stayed in touch after *Buddy* ended in 2002, and had managed to get together once or twice, and had even both worked on projects for the same theatre production company again during the intervening years.

In a way, he was returning a favour by visiting me. Back in 1997, Paul had suffered a heart attack during an audition process, and was admitted to the Chelsea and Westminster Hospital for a bypass operation. While he was there, I paid him a visit. Now, almost twenty years later, here he was to see me.

Unfortunately, our time together was cut short as a hospital porter arrived unexpectedly to take me for a CT scan. But it was wonderful to have an unscheduled visitor, and for the chance to catch up once more.

Paul has a wonderful choreographer wife in Rosita, and their son, Kiyia, has just joined the entertainments team at a resort in Aviemore, Scotland, where I'm sure he'll excel and have a great time into the bargain.

Paul is also the provider of the greatest one-liner I have *ever* heard...

At the end of each year in *Buddy*, usually around September time, there would be a partial cast chance. Some members of the cast would leave, others would stay - and we would spend several weeks rehearsing with the new folk during the day, while performing with the old team each evening. It was usually a fun time, where we got to hang out when not working on stage, camped out in the auditorium and drinking the entire West End's supply of tea and coffee.

One of the wonderful aspects of *Buddy* is that it was considered a 'play with music', rather than a standard musical show. This was down to the fact that no-one stopped mid-sentence to sing about how they were feeling or what was about to happen, such as they might do in *Miss Saigon*, or *Oliver* and other similar productions. The music in *Buddy* came from the characters - such as Buddy Holly and the Crickets - performing the songs they were famous for.

The cast was made up of actor/musicians; everything was played live. No-one ever mimed to playing an instrument or singing (for those interested, I played banjo, percussion and harmonica in the show, and occasionally guitar and/or mandolin when playing my understudy roles).

The show started with a traditional country and western band - The Hayriders - play and sing 'Rose of Texas' before stepping aside for newcomers Buddy, Joe and Jerry to begin playing a similar country number, then get into trouble for launching into an up-tempo rock 'n' roll song instead. This was all went out live on the local radio station, KDAV (still a genuine station in Lubbock, Texas that you can listen to online!) and demonstrated that Buddy wasn't averse to breaking the rules to pursue his love of this new style of music.

As 'Rose of Texas' was the first song to be performed in the show, it had to be good so as to set the tone for what was to come. It would be the first thing the audience heard, after all.

I was a member of The Hayriders during my time in *Buddy*, and learned to play the banjo for that one particular song. Every year, when new actors joined the cast, we would get together in our new line up with the musical director and practice the song and our individual harmonies until we had it note-perfect. Or, as note perfect as we could get it. There was a short, solo banjo riff at the end of the song that I would fluff from time to time, much to the amusement of the other cast members. For a while, it got to be something I dreaded as it approached at each performance - which, of course, made it more certain than not that I was going to screw it up. Ah, well...

Rehearsals would begin with a process known as blocking. This is where the director - Paul Mills - would show the new cast members the basics of where to stand, where to enter and exit, how he wanted their lines performed, and so on. Once the show was blocked, we moved on to include the songs we'd been rehearsing in other parts of the theatre.

Paul returned to work after his heart attack in time for new cast rehearsals to begin, and he had been warned to take things very easily. After a week or so, we came to the day when the new Hayriders line-up would play 'Rose of Texas' for him for the very first time. As we were still in the early days of playing and singing together, let's just say our performance wasn't that great.

As soon as we'd finished, we heard "Stop there!" shouted from out in the auditorium, and we stood watching, silently, as Paul approached. He slowly climbed the steps that led up to the stage and stopped in front of us, stern-faced. After a moment, he spoke, saying the words I will never forget...

"Four surgeons battled for six hours to save my life, so I could listen to *that*."

The man is a legend.

I was allowed home again a few days after my CT scan. Mr Morar and my other doctors were still unable to find out why I was coughing up blood, and that particular nastiness was gradually receding of its own volition.

So, with no real answers, I returned home once again (many thanks to Lauren Corless for kindly bringing Kirsty to collect me), and I tried to restart my rest and recuperation all over again.

A TARGET FOR TOMMY

By now, you will undoubtedly be aware of several facts, including...

- I was in hospital a lot.
- I was frequently bored.
- I read a lot to fill the time.
- I really like *Doctor Who*.

So, imagine my excitement when I discovered what my friend Paul Magrs had done now. He was the one who had arranged the amazing message from Russell T Davies, and a fantastic writer. Do yourself a favour and read Paul's books as soon as you can. My favourites are his *Brenda & Effie* adventures!

Paul had contacted a mutual friend of ours, Stuart Douglas. Stuart is the owner of *Obverse Books*, an Edinburgh based publisher that produces a vast range of incredible titles from books featuring Paul's *Doctor Who* spin-off character, *Iris Wildthyme* to critical explorations of classic sci-fi TV series, and much more.

Together, they hatched a plan...

During the original classic era of *Doctor Who*, it was rare for episodes to be repeated on TV and, if they ever were, it was normally after a considerable amount of time had passed. With no such thing as video tapes or DVDs for most of the show's history, this meant that if you missed a story - you missed a story, and had to hope that the BBC would one day see fit to show it again.

One lifeline were the novelisations of the stories, issued by a publishing imprint called *Target Books*. In 1973, they began to publish these slim volumes, often with one of the TV writers, such as the great Terrence Dicks, as the author. The books were not only a way to 're-watch' your favourite adventures and catch up on those you had missed, but they frequently delved deeper into the story's characters, making them hugely popular with *Doctor Who* fans worldwide.

What Paul and Stuart decided to do was to write and publish a limited edition, faux *Target* book, filled with brand new *Doctor Who* stories written especially for me! This book, called *A Target For Tommy* was to be written by some of my favourite writers and friends, including Philip Ardagh, Paul Cornell, Daniel Blythe, Roy Gill, Sharon Tregenza, Steve Cole, Barry Hutchison and Paul Magrs himself. My apologies to anyone I've left off that list; I didn't miss you out on purpose!

What's more, the profits from the book would be donated to me to help support my family during this particularly difficult time. How amazing is that? To say I was honoured is a vast understatement!

The day my first copy arrived is one I will remember for as long as I live. Paul had drawn the cover himself, and every story contained inside was utterly brilliant. I'm so incredibly proud and thankful to everyone involved for all their hard work. And not only were the tales of time and space wonderful to read, the financial help that shortly followed went a long way to making my family's life better at a time when I was unable to work.

As *A Target For Tommy* had a limited release, chances are you probably won't be able to get hold of a copy now, making the ones currently out there precious prize possessions. However, you may be able to take a peek at the cover if you search for the title online.

Once again, thank you to everyone involved in this special project, especially to Paul Magrs and Stuart Douglas. I'm blessed to have such good friends.

BEDDY BYES

To sleep, perchance to dream.

I don't do a lot of either, these days. Although that is now gradually changing.

Because I find it difficult to use the stairs (and because I don't want to take any further tumbles), I've been sleeping in the living room, using my armchair and foot stool as a surprisingly serviceable bed. Plus, it allows me to prop myself up at night, which helps with both my breathing, and my recovery.

Then, recently, the district nurse explained that the NHS can provide me with a hospital bed for the living room. I wasn't sure at first. When my Dad became too ill to sit and sleep in his armchair, he had a hospital bed set up in his living room. He was very reluctant to use it at first because - as he said to me, he knew that once he got into it, he wouldn't get back out again.

Obviously, my situation is different, but his words were playing on my mind.

Eventually, I agreed and an adjustable hospital bed was delivered and set up in the living room for me. It included an inflatable mattress that would mould to me body, and allow me to be comfortable for extended periods of time. It was connected to a pump that would add and remove just the right amount of air as I moved around during the night.

Or so they claimed.

What actually happened was that the mattress slowly deflated during the night, leaving me lying on the metal bars of the frame below. In essence, the exact opposite of comfort. Whatever crazy word that might be.

The engineer returned on several occasions to reset the pump and make sure that it was working correctly. Both times, he assured me that yes, it was.

And, both times, I ended up trying to sleep on metal bars.

Eventually, I gave up and asked for a normal mattress. One that didn't require a computer operated pump connected to it in order for me to sleep. I know, such a bizarre concept, eh? One was duly provided, and I've been sleeping better and better every night since.

What's wonderful is the ability to use the control pad to adjust the height of the bed and the headrest to ensure I'm in the most comfortable position. I no longer had to rely on a stack of pillows staying in place all night.

Plus, if I felt wiped out or unwell during the day - which I occasionally do - I'm able to hop into the bed for a quick nap.

Or at least, I was - until Sam discovered the control pad.

Instantly, the bed became less of a bed, and more of an exciting piece of training equipment for potential astronauts. Many's the time when I would hear the whirring of motors, and he would gradually rise up over the back of the sofa, sitting rigidly upright, and holding a smart salute.

Then, without so much as a smirk, he'd press another button, and he'd slowly descend from view.

By which time, I'd usually be in fits of laughter.

I found the ritual of bedtime less funny, however. I've mentioned previously that I struggled to cope with the gradual repositioning of the family upstairs each evening. First the boys would go up to play on their respective games consoles - Arran doing so the split second the final mouthful of his dinner had passed his lips. Sam liked to stay down for a while to spend time with me and Kirsty but, before too long, he too would head up to his room.

Last to go would be Kirsty, followed dutifully by our two dogs, Ruby and Pixie. Leaving yours truly alone until the morning.

After all those weeks in hospital, including several in a room by myself, you would think I'd be used to being by myself at night. But I didn't find it easy. In part because I was hit by bouts of loneliness and feeling down, but also because I found it difficult to call out to Kirsty if I needed any help.

To rectify the situation, Kirsty has now made the decision to begin sleeping downstairs with me to keep me company. She sleeps on one of the sofas, which she professes to be perfectly comfortable. (It true, they are).

She's a keeper, that one!

SUE AND BRYAN

There are two important members of my family that I haven't introduced you to, yet - my sister, Sue, and my brother, Bryan.

Sue was born a few years after me and I clearly remember the day my parents brought her home from the hospital, even though I was still a toddler.

Our first meeting didn't go that well...

MUM: "Tommy, we'd like you to meet your new baby sister, Jayne..."

I looked down at the tiny baby, wrapped up in her blankets.

ME: "I don't want a Jayne."

DAD: "What?"

ME: "I said, I don't want a Jayne. I want a Susan."

MUM: "Don't be silly. This is your sister, Jayne."

ME: "You're not listening to me... I don't want a Jayne. Take it back wherever you found it, and get a Susan instead!"

My Mum and Dad assured each other that I would come round to their way of thinking in the end.

But, I didn't.

I called the baby 'Susan' at every opportunity.

Until, eventually, my parents changed my sister's name to Susan Jayne Donbavand.

A year later, I'd started school – and my best friend in class, Ellis, just happened to live across the road from me.

After school, we used to go to a little play park along the street. You know the kind of thing – a couple of swings, a slide, a roundabout. Both my Mum and Ellis's Mum could see the park from our houses, so it was all perfectly safe.

Then came the half-term holiday – and it rained. All week.

I was stuck inside, and SO bored!

Eventually, on the Sunday afternoon, the rain stopped and I begged my Mum to let me play out with Ellis.

Eventually, she agreed, telling me to be careful. So, I called for Ellis, and we went down to the park.

But we couldn't play on any of the equipment – everything was soaking wet. We were especially disappointed that we couldn't use the slide. It was long, made of metal, and went really fast.

But it had also sat out in the rain all week, and was still soaking.

So, I told Ellis to wait there while I went to get something I could use to dry the slide. I ran home and searched everywhere – considering borrowing a tea towel, unravelling reams of toilet paper, and so on.

Until I saw the perfect thing I could use to dry the slide...

...my baby sister!

No, think about it! She was wrapped up in all her blankets, and she was wearing a nappy – she'd make a perfect sponge!

So, I waited until my Mum wasn't looking – and then, I kidnapped my sister.

Back at the park, Ellis waited at the bottom of the slide, while I pushed my sister up the steps, and then – WHOOSH!

She went like a rocket!

Straight through Ellis's legs at the bottom.

It was OK, though; she stopped when she hit the fence.

And, it had worked! She slide was now dryer than before.

We spent the next twenty minutes pushing my baby sister down a wet slide until my Mum looked out of the widow and realised what we were doing.

I *may* have got into trouble.

Several years later, my brother, Bryan, was born. I didn't try to change his name, but I did cry when I found out he was a boy as it meant I'd have to share a bedroom and Sue could keep one by herself.

When Bryan was around two years old, I was 11 - and we devised a game called 'Knock Out', after we'd seen our Dad watching some big boxing match on TV. Obviously, we didn't really box - we just pretended and, taking it in turns, one of us would pretend to be knocked out. Then, the other would shout "Knock out!", and parade around the room, basking in the glory of the win.

Then came Christmas morning...

Bryan woke up before me, very excited, and came running over to my bed (yes, we shared a room!) to get me up. He shook me, shouting something along the lines of, "Tommygetupit'sChristmasgetupgetupgetup!"

I was still half asleep, and hadn't yet realised the significance of the day. To my tired mind, Bryan was waking me up to play 'Knock Out'. So, without even opening my eyes, I lifted up the bed sheets, and...

SMASH!

I punched my two year old brother straight in the face.

To give Bryan his credit, he was so stunned that he didn't start crying until around 20 seconds later. Sadly, 20 seconds wasn't quite long enough for me to find somewhere to hide from my parents for the rest of my life, and again, I *may* have got into a little trouble.

These days, both Bryan and Sue have families of their own. Sue is married to Kev, with teen twins Aoife and Luke, and younger Noah.

Bryan married Bridget a few years ago, and they have our immediate family's newest arrival, Eliza.

I love them all to bits.

And I know that my brother and sister are there for me, whenever I need them. Just as I am for both of them.

Although, I'm too scared to play 'Knock Out' with either of them.

IN REMISSION

mazing news...

I'm in remission!

I've just returned from an appointment with Dr Biswas. He had studied the results of my latest round of scans and tests and announced the good news that there is no longer any sign of my cancer.

I'm so happy, and will admit that tears were shed in the ENT department of Blackburn Hospital for the second time, albeit for a very different reason.

I'm finding it very difficult to put my whirling emotions into words, so this will most likely be quite a short update. Of course, I know that I'm not cured, and that the cancer may yet return, but - for now at least - I beat the bastard!

WHOOSH!

Oh dear.

I thought the good news was too good to last.

Don't worry - it's not another health scare, and I haven't been admitted to back into hospital (for a change).

This 'oh dear' is down to work...

I LOVE my job. Writing full time is a dream come true, and one which I've been lucky enough to do for over ten years now.

I quit my day job on 30th September, 2006. How can I be so sure of the date? Easy - it's the day my son, Sam, was born.

Whoa! Wait a minute! I hear some of you cry. (Go on, open the window and cry it out of there. You don't know where I live, it *might* just work.) *You resigned from a full-time job on the day your son was born?*

Yep. I agree that, under normal circumstances, that wouldn't be a very wise decision and, should you ever find yourself in a similar situation, I urge you to spend time seriously contemplating the choice before you jump.

However, it was the right decision for me and my family. I'd already written several books, and had been contracted to ghost-write for a new kids series called *Too Ghoul For School* which was published under the pen name, B. Strange.

Plus, I already had a good number of school visits booked (my first ever!), and there were more coming in all the time.

Soon afterwards, I had an amazing literary agent (Hi, Penny!), and I was to get my first big publishing deal - the one with Walker Books to write *Scream Street*.

Fast forward to now, and school visits are out of the question, cutting off a large part of my income. That leaves me with just writing as a way to earn money and support my family, and I've already had to turn down several projects in that field due to my illness.

Until recently, I've found the familiar act of sitting at my computer and writing very difficult to do. A combination of constantly feeling tired, and quickly aching whenever I sit up at a desk, have made the actual process almost impossible.

That's not to say I haven't had work to do. A few weeks before I was diagnosed, I was commissioned to write a new kids horror series for Oxford University Press (OUP) called *The Creeper Files*. This series would also be written under a fake name - Hacker Murphy - who was to be the investigative reporter looking into claims that a half-man, half-plant creature was terrorising the small town of Larkspur and its residents. Three brave kids - Jake, Liam and Sarah - would be at the forefront of each of the four 30,000 word adventures.

I was really looking forward to writing the series, and was around two-thirds of the way through the first book - *The Root of All Evil* - when I was given the bad news about my cancer.

I tried to continue work on the book once my treatment began, but it soon became clear that I wasn't going to be able to continue. The deadlines given for submitting each draft of a book are extremely important in the publishing industry, and especially in this case as OUP had already scheduled dates in their future catalogue for the books to come out.

Obviously, there are times when missing a deadline is impossible to avoid, even for the most experienced writers. The late, great Douglas Adams, author of *The Hitchhiker's Guide to the Galaxy*, once famously said:

"I love deadlines. I love the whooshing noise they make as they go by."

But, the last thing an author wants is get a reputation for missing deadlines and submitting work late. If that should happen, it won't just be deadlines that 'whoosh' as they fly past, it will be job opportunities as well.

By now, I was late with the first draft of *The Root of All Evil*, and I had to admit to my editor that I was struggling to finish the manuscript.

To some, the obvious option may have been to either cancel the series outright, or at least postpone it until I was well enough to get back to work again. However, OUP had, by now, paid me the advance for the books and neither they, nor I, liked the idea of my having to pay it all back. Not that I could, as I was barely earning at this stage.

So, the publishers took the unusual step of finding another writer who could step in to finish book one, and write the second book in the series, *Welcome to the Jungle*. And who did they choose but my good friend and the person providing you with updates on my condition earlier in this book, Barry Hutchison!

I was thrilled, and the situation was interesting enough for the publishing industry's magazine, *The Bookseller*, asked us to write an article about it. I've copied and pasted that article as the next chapter so you can read it for yourself.

Then it came time for me to write the final two titles in *The Creeper Files* series - *Terror from the Taps*, and *Incy, Wincy Eek!* By now, I was stronger, and sure I would be able to work my way through the 30,000 words required in time to meet the deadline.

I wasn't.

Once again, I was late submitting the book, and the publishers have now decided that Barry will go on to write the fourth instalment instead of me.

I'm obviously disappointed, but especially with myself as I've come to realise that I wasn't being honest, with my editor or my agent - but, especially with myself.

I'm not yet strong enough to sit down and write an entire book. I simply can't write as quickly, or for as long as I used to be able to, and I can't continue to take on large projects until I am able to once more.

That said, I'm thrilled that Barry and I have finally been able to collaborate on a series of books, even if it didn't happen in the way that either of us had ever envisaged it.

Now, please turn the page to read the article Barry and I wrote about our unique situation for *The Bookseller*, and please seek out the four books in the fantastic series *The Creeper Files*, now that you know who the author, Hacker Murphy, really is!

CREEPING TOGETHER

T*his was the article Barry and I wrote together for The Bookseller magazine about our experience of working on The Creeper Files.*

In March 2016, children's author, Tommy Donbavand, was diagnosed with cancer. Intensive treatment left him in intensive care, unable to work on *The Creeper Files*, a series of books he had been commissioned to write for Oxford University Press.

With deadlines and publishing slots looming, and Tommy unavailable, Tommy's friend and fellow children's author, Barry Hutchison, received an urgent call.

TD: Early in 2016, I went undercover. After writing almost 100 children's books of my own, I now had a secret identity. Thanks to the team at OUP, I was Hacker Murphy, investigative reporter on the trail of a terrifying half-man, half-plant beast known only as The Creeper.

I enjoyed my new identity, and plunged into writing the first of four adventures in the series, *The Root of All Evil*.

I was around just over half way through the first draft when I was diagnosed with inoperable throat cancer. Rigorous courses of both chemotherapy and radiotherapy swiftly followed, leaving me unwell, and fatigued.

A week later, I was rushed into critical care unconscious, and suffering from double pneumonia and sepsis. I remained in hospital for over a month.

When I eventually arrived home, I found it increasingly difficult to sit up at my desk and write and, with deadlines looming, the pressure was on. I didn't want to bring the entire series to a halt at such an early stage.

BH: And that's where I stepped in. Tommy and I first 'met' back at the tail end of the 90s, via an online writing community. We've been in contact pretty much every day since.

We share the same sense of humour, and are sounding boards for each other as we develop new book ideas. I was even best man at Tommy's wedding, and spent most of my speech plugging my books.

It was Tommy who first suggested I try writing for children, and in many ways I owe my entire career to him. So, when Tommy's agent and editor got in touch to ask if I'd be prepared to take on some of his workload, I jumped at the chance to help him out.

The first manuscript was half-written, the second one plotted out. I'd discussed the storyline with Tommy in one of our regular Skype sessions before he took ill, so I was familiar enough with the characters and plot to just chuck myself into the writing.

It felt odd at first, working through that first book. I felt like an interloper sneaking through a friend's house and rummaging in their sock drawer when they were out. I didn't change any of Tommy's text on the first draft, and the manuscript I ended up with was a deformed, Frankenstein's monster of a thing with the stitching clearly visible. It wasn't until draft two, after Tommy reassured me via text – he couldn't speak by that point – that I was able to smooth over the joins.

TD: The stress was eased, and I couldn't have been happier that Barry – a good friend, and a very talented writer – had been chosen to take over the series for a while. He finished book one, and wrote book two, *Welcome to the Jungle*, with such skill that I defy anyone to spot the join. I'm now working hard to complete the third book in The Creeper Files series, *Terror from the Taps*.

NOT A CHRISTMAS CRACKER

To paraphrase the late, great John Lennon...
> *And so, that was Christmas*
> *But, what did you eat?*

Man, I love me some Christmas dinner!

It's the King of all dinners. You can even have a turkey crown! (Wahey!)

Kirsty makes the roast dinners to end all roast dinners. Her roast potatoes, in particular, are incredible. Plus, she always cooks sprouts and parsnips - even though I'm the only one in the family who eats either of them!

But, as many of you will know, I've been unable to eat any kind of solid food since the middle of May. Don't get me wrong - I'm trying - and I've even managed a few teaspoons of soup here and there. But, anything more solid is a no go.

So, last Sunday, I had to sit and (try not to) watch as Kirsty and the boys tucked into their roast turkey with all the trimmings.

I had a few tropical flavour milkshakes to pour down my stomach tube.

We tried blending some turkey, potato and gravy for the

tube, but that didn't work. It was either too thick, or ended up a warm, brown water.

I will admit to ending up in tears.

Not because I'm greedy, or was jealous of my own family (they genuinely offered not to have Christmas dinner if it was going to upset me, but I turned that suggestion down flat).

I cried because I am so utterly fed up with being unwell all the bloody time.

It's never ending.

Not a day goes by without some stark reminder that cancer has turned my entire life - and the lives of all those around me - completely upside down.

Whether that's getting a swollen tongue, being in pain with more mouth ulcers, having a coughing fit (blood stained tissues optional), feeling weak, being unable to sleep, being unable to stay awake, high temperatures, hallucinations from said high temperatures - or one of dozens of other long-lasting, ongoing, never sodding going away symptoms of my illness.

And Christmas brought it all to a head.

I've never felt so alone while surrounded by my family as I did last Sunday.

Actually, that's not true. It started in the run up to Christmas (which begins in what, March, now?) I couldn't take part in any Christmas shopping, for example. OK, so I don't enjoy shopping at the best of times, and especially when the shops are packed at this time of year. But I would still like the option to do it, rather than have that choice taken away from me.

I wanted to help out, but simply couldn't.

I was able to pick out presents for the boys, and for my nieces and nephews - but then had to sit out while Kirsty bought them, tested them, inserted batteries, wrapped them, etc.

Plus, having now not worked for almost ten months, this ended up being a very slender Christmas for us, as you might imagine.

We couldn't get the boys everything they'd wanted, or that we wanted to get for them. Not that we ever go overboard, or simply buy them everything on their lists - but this year we had to compromise and economise more than we've ever had to before.

That's a crappy feeling. Especially because both boys were so amazingly understanding about it when we explained it to them in the run up to the big day.

Cue tears, again. Mine, not theirs.

One thing we always look forward to is decorating the Christmas tree. Kirsty usually puts the tree up and adds the lights, then the boys go to town on the decorations while I play a selection of seasonal songs and supervise. Then we switch to karaoke versions of the tracks and have a good old Christmas sing-a-long in the newly twinkling lights.

Guess what?

Because I'm still sleeping in my NHS hospital bed in the living room, we didn't have enough room for our usual tree. Not unless we could somehow get rid of the bed and I found a way to nest in the lower branches each night.

So - compromise time again - we picked up a smaller, table top tree which the boys were able to decorate before Noddy Holder had time to screech...

"It's Chriiiiissssssttmmaaaaassss!"

I switched over to the karaoke tracks, but I couldn't speak the words, let alone sing them. After a few goes each, the boys went to their bedrooms to play on their games consoles and I switched off the music.

On Christmas morning, I like to video proceedings for future viewing, always starting the footage as I head downstairs to 'see if Father Christmas has been'. I can't do stairs anymore, so had to film the unwrapping from the armchair where I now spend a good 75% of my life. Not a big change, I know, but another little reminder that things were different this year.

And that wasn't the end of it.

A wee dram to celebrate the big day? Nope. A sneaky mince pie as I put one out for Santa? No chance. Going for a potter around heavily-laden stalls of the Christmas market? Not a hope.

A nibble on Rudolph's carrot? Not since the court case and restraining order...

Sigh!

Despite the changes to our usual festivities, Kirsty and the boys threw themselves into the fun and had a great time. And I really wish that I had been able to do the same - but I just couldn't.

All I could think about was how I'd caused this. Not purposefully, of course. I know that. But, everyone was having to make sacrifices because I can't fight off the effects of this cancer shit.

And I hated the fact that I was potentially going to spoil it all for them by feeling this way!

Now, I know what you're saying - that I shouldn't be thinking like that, and that it isn't my fault at all, and how everything will be back to normal next year...

Except - I'm not sure that it will be any better next year. Or the year after that.

I'm starting to become convinced that this is as good as I'm going to get. That I simply won't get any better than this.

It does happen to some cancer patients; they never fully recover the ability to eat or speak.

That's if I'm still here for another Christmas.

And, let me tell you, that's a jolly thought to flash across your mind as you watch your kids unwrap their presents.

The cancer could easily return and, the longer this all goes on for, the more certain I am that that's exactly what will happen.

By then, all I could think about is how awful the family's Christmas would be if the worst did come to the worst.

Cue: more tears.

So, that was my Christmas 2016. It's almost over, thank goodness; tomorrow is New Year's Eve, when I once again won't be able to celebrate with anything more exotic than a tasteless milkshake or three.

I'm not sure whether to look forward to 2017 or not. It surely can't be any worse than this year has been.

Please believe me, I'm really trying not to feel sorry for myself. I just wasn't expecting Christmas to hit home quite so hard.

Thanks - as ever - for reading and putting up with my self-obsessed ranting. I'll try to post something a little more positive next time.

WEIGHT AND SEE

I n an earlier chapter, I discussed the fact that having cancer has caused me to lose weight. I'd like to return to that topic, if I may...

When I was first diagnosed with cancer, I was the fattest I had ever been. Kirsty didn't used like me using the word 'fat', preferring instead to call me 'large' or 'weighty'. But, the truth of the matter is, I was fat.

I've struggled with my weight since my late 20s. I was never fat because of food (no sweet tooth, remember - so no cakes, crisps, sweets, etc.), but I did have a penchant for cheese. Lots of cheese!

I also drank alcohol, often in the places where I worked, such as the holiday camps and cruise liners. I didn't drink excessively, but it was clearly enough that it made a difference.

Then, after I left acting to become a writer, I spent most of each day sitting in a chair, working. This didn't help at all and, by March 2016, I weighed 22 stone 4 (or 312 pounds for readers across the pond).

Being so overweight probably contributed to my cancer

developing, and it was clear that something had to be done. And something was done, but not what I ever expected. I lost the ability to eat solid food.

That happened, you may recall, on 1st May 2016. From that day to the present, I've 'eaten' by pouring NHS provided milkshakes into my stomach via a rubber tube. With the best will in the world, it's impossible to maintain the same calorie intake when using this method, and so I began to lose weight.

And I didn't stop losing weight. To the point where my doctors, and especially my nutritionist, Cara, started to become concerned.

Each bottle of milkshake provides me with 300 calories, and the doctors wanted me to 'drink' six of these a day, providing me with a grand total of 1,800 of the little charmers. As the recommended calorie intake for men is around 2,500 in order to maintain weight, dropping to 1,800 would help me to gradually lose weight.

However, I quickly found that if I had too many milkshakes, I became ill and brought them back up, completely defeating the purpose of the exercise. At best, I could manage four milkshakes a day and, on some days, could only stomach two.

That's either 600 or 1,200 calories per day. Not enough.

And so, the weight dropped off me far too quickly. You'll probably be aware that it simply isn't healthy to lose weight too fast, not that I was particularly healthy to be begin with during this time.

To try to remedy the situation, the last time I was in hospital my bottles of milkshake were replaced with a large bag of the stuff that was fed into my stomach peg by an electric pump that I had to carry with me whenever I wanted to get in or out of bed, or visit the bathroom.

This pumped milkshake directly into my system for 18 hours at a time. Yep, that's not a typo - it took 18 straight hours to pump an entire bag of this goop into me, then I was allowed a couple of hours off before a fresh bag was attached.

This had the effect of causing me to swell like a balloon, and vomit regularly.

Not ideal.

So, after a few days, I was allowed to go back to manually pouring bottles of the stuff into my system, with the promise that I would do my best to keep to four a day at the very minimum. I was also given pots of 'calorie shots' that would add to my intake without causing me too much discomfort.

I have, to the most part, kept up my regime of four bottles and two shots per day, unless I've been unwell with a stomach bug or similar virus. That hasn't stopped the weight loss, though and - as I write this - I now weigh in at just 9 stone 4 (128 pounds). That means I've lost just over 13 stones (184 pounds).

I know.

As a result, I don't look good. I resemble a badly wrapped skeleton, covered with loose, saggy skin.

Until recently, I'd been restricted to washing myself by hand in the bathroom downstairs. Eventually, I really wanted a shower, and asked Kirsty and Arran to help me upstairs. It was tough, but we made it.

Once in the main bathroom, I saw myself in a full length mirror for the first time in months. The shock of what I now look like was so severe that I broke down and cried for several hours.

I'm gradually becoming used to looking like this, and being so weak as a result of losing so much weight so quickly. And it's now another problem I will have to tackle if and when I ever emerge from this seemingly endless ordeal.

THAT'S JUST SWELL

O K, so it appears nature has decided I'm not quite ill enough. And so, it has arranged for me to develop lymphedema.

Lymphedema is a condition where certain lymph nodes in your body don't drain fluid as they should, a situation that is frequently caused by bouts of radiotherapy. Lucky me, eh?

We have lymph nodes all over our bodies and, when they malfunction, the fluid remains in the surrounding flesh, casing painful swelling. For me, this has happened in my throat and neck which, coupled with my skeletal frame thanks to excessive weight loss, makes me look like I have a massive sodding head.

Not only that, but the swollen areas continue to make it difficult for me to swallow and, therefore eat, drink and talk.

Thankfully, the good old NHS has treatment available, but it's nothing like I had been expecting.

In order to help drain the areas of fluid, a trained nurse gently massages and strokes the affected areas, and shines a powerful infrared torch onto my skin. Going to a medical centre in Accrington twice a week for a massage and a bit of a glow is an unusual state of affairs, but that's exactly what happens. The course of treatment lasts for three to six weeks, and I've just finished my first go around. I'm now waiting to hear the dates of my second course.

In between sessions, I have a special head mask to wear that provides mild compression to the affected areas and, as a welcome side effect, makes me look like a Mexican wrestler.

Not sure what my name should be, though. How does *El Authoro* grab you?

UPDATE: Yay! I not only have lymphedema, but I also now suffer from trismus!

What's that? Never heard of it? No, neither had I. I was forced to look it up with the use of everybody's friendly neighbourhood search engine, Google.

And, guess what? Trismus is a form of lockjaw!

Hurray!

sigh

Yes, thanks to a combination of the lymphedema, radio-therapy and general ill health, I can now only open my mouth a centimetre or so. Even if I was able to eat, I'd have to restrict my diet to thin foods, like strips of bacon, raw lasagne sheets, and floppy disks.

And what's the treatment for trismus, I hear you ask? Why, it's being measured for a gadget that I clamp between my teeth and gradually widen for force my upper and lower jaws apart over an extended period of time.

I can't wait!

TALK TALK

Admission time...

I've been on anti-depressant medication for several years now. It all started around the time that the West End show I was in was closing, and I was about to lose the best job I'd ever had. I found myself increasingly wanting to hide away; I stopped socialising with my friends and couldn't bear being around strangers. On the rare occasion that I did go out in public, such as to travel to and from the theatre where I worked, I started to get angry and shout at strangers if they behaved in a way I considered inappropriate. That wasn't like me at all.

After a while, I only really spoke to my brother, Bryan, who lived with me in London. I just couldn't bring myself to be more outgoing and open.

Then, a good friend of mine, Gus, was given the task of providing the kilometre markers for a charity 10k run. Being an incredibly gifted musician himself, he came up with the idea of placing a busker at the end of each one kilometre stage, playing as the participants ran by. He called and asked if I would busk with my harmonica at one of these stages.

The thought terrified me, and I ended up in floods of tears. Bryan didn't know how to help, other than to say he was going for a walk and that he wanted me to telephone The Samaritans while he was out. I tried to make excuses, insisting that I wasn't about to hurt myself in any way, but he insisted. So I did.

The person I spoke to was wonderful. She suggested that it sounded as if my doctor would be a good person to turn to. As soon as I hung up, I called to make an appointment.

A few days later, the doctor explained that depression was an imbalance of chemicals in the brain, and not just a case of 'feeling down' and he prescribed an ongoing course of anti-depressants to help correct that disparity. It took a week or so, but they soon began to help and the world brightened considerably.

Since then, I've coped reasonably well, and was even in the process of gradually stepping down my medication with a view to eventually stop taking it.

Then, I was diagnosed with cancer.

This was, as you can imagine, not only a terrible situation for my physical well-being, but it was also a major blow to my mental health. The ensuing cancer treatment, their side effects and a lengthy stay in hospital only served to make the situation worse.

I found myself feeling really down in a way I hadn't experienced since my brother urged me to seek help all those years ago. Once again, I wasn't in any way going to harm myself, but there were days that I could simply not see the point of going on. If someone had told me that when I closed my eyes that night I would never open them again, I would not have argued with them.

Kirsty encouraged me to talk about these feelings to the district nurse during her next visit, which I did. She was as wonderful as I'd come to expect, and referred me to the local counselling service for help. After a short while, I was given the date to begin a course of therapy.

My counsellor, Janet, has been amazing. Talking with her has helped me in so many ways, and I'm now feeling much more positive, brighter and almost back to my old self again.

At first, I found the venue for my counselling sessions - the local hospice - a little unsettling. But I soon got used to it, even if my throat didn't.

I found that, following each hour long session, I would cough up blood from my throat for a while. I initially put this down to the fact that I was doing lots of talking - something I hadn't done for quite a while due to the pain and discomfort I was in. But then I realised that my throat began to bleed while I was sitting in the waiting room, before my appointments with Janet had even started!

It was Kirsty who worked out what was going on. In order to establish a calming atmosphere, the hospice used essential oils and aromatherapy. This was what was affecting my throat and causing it to bleed!

I've now completed my scheduled course of counselling sessions, but the option is there for more, should I feel the need for them.

If you or a loved one ever find yourself in a situation where counselling is required, I urge you to give it a go. The results can be truly remarkable.

ONWARDS AND UPWARDS

Well, that's about it.

The book, I mean, not my recuperation. That still has quite a way to go yet.

The date today is Sunday, 9th July 2017, and I'm busy putting the final touches to this book. It will be published in four days' time, on Thursday 13th, and I'm thrilled to say that over 120 people have already pre-ordered a copy.

If you're currently reading the ebook version of *Tommy V Cancer*, you may be interested to know that I'm planning to create a paperback book. Check back to Amazon now and again, and you should see it pop up soon.

If you're reading that paperback, you already know!

You may now know, however, that I'm also planning an audiobook version, read by yours truly. Yes, I do still struggle with my speech a little, but I've made a conscious effort to be open and honest all throughout my journey, and letting you hear how I currently sound will continue that trend.

Now, are you ready for some incredible news?

I'm now one year cancer free!

I'm so thrilled, and so are my friends, family and even

many strangers. There were times when I genuinely believed I wouldn't get this far. But, I have, and I intend to continue that way.

Plus, breaking news - as of four or five days ago, I'm able to drink again! It literally happened overnight. I went to bed still struggling to take sips of water, and woke up able to drink a whole bottle of the stuff!

I can only hope that the ability to eat appears in the same way. My doctors have suggested that it will be around another four years before I am completely recovered and can say that I have finally beaten my cancer, so there's a long road ahead of me.

But I know I'll be walking it with Kirsty, Arran, Sam, Sue, Bryan and everyone else who is special to me. This is a horrible journey to undertake, but you don't have to do it alone.

With that in mind, there are certain people I would like to thank for their unending care, support and love...

My wife, Kirsty, of course - without whom, I doubt I would be here to be writing these very words. I love you with all my heart.

My sons, Sam and Arran. You guys mean the whole world to me, and much more besides. It is an honour to play a part in helping you to become amazing young men. I love you both.

My sister Sue, and brother Bryan. You've always been there for me, even when it was scary and difficult to do so. We've been through a lot together, and there will be more to come. I love you both, and everyone in your own families - Kev,

Bridget, Aoife, Luke, Noah and Eliza (as well as future family additions we've yet to meet).

My Mum and Dad, whose love and upbringing made me the person I am today. I miss you both like crazy, but know you've both been watching over me every step of the way.

My extended family - Marie, Phil, Shelagh, Roy, Les, Lyn, John, Janette, and everyone else. It would take an entire second book to name you all, and I don't have time to write that. It's meant so much to me knowing you're always ready to help me with anything I need.

My amazing pal, Barry. We may not get to see each in other in person very often, but you're always on the other end of an online chat. The help and support you've given me through all this has been incredible.

Mr Morar, Dr Biswas, Cara, Sharron, Emma, Lucy, Mairi and all the doctors, nurses, radiographers, chemo specialists and staff who have looked after me so amazingly since this nightmare began, and will continue to do so. As my Dad once said, I've met angels, but they were in disguise.

Huge thanks to Nigel Parkinson, the legend behind the art for my great *Beano* characters, including *Dennis the Menace*, for the amazing cover illustration and artwork on the *Tommy V Cancer* website.

To everyone who works tirelessly to rid the world of cancer, you're my hero.

And, finally, to you. My friends – now, old, online or real life. And even the total strangers who have reached out with their prayers and good wishes. It really does mean so much to me.

If I've missed anyone out, it was not done deliberately. Thank you so much for taking the time to read my story. If you or someone you know or love is either going through their own battle, or is about to do so, I hope that my words have helped you to understand and prepare for what lies ahead. If that is the case, please take all my good thoughts with you. If you're not connected to anyone fighting this terrible disease, I hope I managed to raise a smile.

Tommy Donbavand
9th July, 2017

TOMMY'S BOOKS

W hat follows is a list of my currently available books. All of these titles are available in the UK, with many published in the US, and other countries.

In the UK: http://amzn.to/2ueY6TJ
In the US: http://amzn.to/2t12OEm

Scream Street series:
Fang of the Vampire
Blood of the Witch
Heart of the Mummy
Flesh of the Zombie
Skull of the Skeleton
Claw of the Werewolf
Invasion of the Normals
Attack of the Trolls
Terror of the Nightwatchman
Rampage of the Goblins
Hunger of the Yeti

Secret of the Changeling
Flame of the Dragon
Wail of the Banshee
Gloves of the Ghoulkeeper
Shiver of the Phantom
Negatives Attract
A Sneer Death Experience
Unwanted Guests
Looks Like Trouble

Fangs: Vampire Spy series:
Operation: Golden Bum
Codename: The Tickler
Assignment: Royal Rescue
Target: Nobody, Walker Books
Project: Wolf World
Mission: Lullaby

Snow-Man series:
Hot Hot Hot!
Stone Age!
What A Drip!
Windy-Pops!
It's A Gas!
Cold Front!
Hot! Hot! Hot! The Play

Space Hoppers series:
Mudmen from Mars
Silence on Saturn
Undead of Uranus

Nursery on Neptune
Victory for Venus
Panic on Pluto
Jailbreak on Jupiter
Monsters on Mercury
End-Game on Earth

Time Trek series:

Rampage Through Rome
Nightmare Near the Nile
Chaos in Camelot
Emergency for England
Frantic in France
Grief by The Globe
Skirmish at Sea
War Over Waterloo

Doctor Who:

Shroud of Sorrow

Tommy Donbavand's Funny Shorts:

My Granny Bit My Bum
Duck
Night of the Toddlers
Viking Kong
The Curious Case of the Panicky Parrot
Invasion of Badger's Bottom
Dinner Ladies of Doooooom!
There's a Time Portal in My Pants

Other books:

Princess Frog-Snogger
They Came From Class 6c!
Our Head Teacher is a Super-Villain
Cyber Shock, Collins Educational
The Terrible Tale of Melody Doom
Once Upon a Time
Zombie!
Uniform
Wolf
Virus
Save the Day
The Sand Witch
Blast to the Past
My Teacher Ate My Brain
Home
Kidnap
Ward 13
Dead Scared
Copy Cat
Just Bite
Raven
Annie
Ringtone
The Girl in the Wall
MC Cesar

Graphic novels:

The Head is Dead
The Colony

Non-Fiction:

Shakespeare
Making a Drama Out of a Crisis
Quick Fixes For Bored Kids
More Quick Fixes For Bored Kids
Quick Fixes For Kids' Parties
Boredom Busters
13 Steps to Beating Writers' Block
Tommy V Cancer

Too Ghoul For School Series:
    (Writing as B. Strange)
    Terror in Cubicle Four
    Silent But Deadly
    School Spooks Day
    Attack of the Zombie Nits
    A Fete Worse Than Death

The Creeper Files series:
    (Writing as Hacker Murphy)
    Root of All Evil
    Terror From The Taps

KICK CANCER UP THE ARSE

Ⓘf you enjoyed this book, and would like to help out, please consider making a donation to The Swallows - a wonderful charity supporting Head and Neck Cancer sufferers and survivors.

You can donate using the link below, and choose between a single or monthly donation...

https://www.justgiving.com/theswallows

The Swallows

Registered Charity Number 1149794

Head Office:

The Charity Shop, 68-70 Waterloo Road, South Shore, Blackpool, FY4 1AB

AND FINALLY...

I f you'd like to receive news about forthcoming books, updates to existing titles, details of live events, and info about cool competitions - why not join my mailing list? Just click on the link below, enter your email address, and you'll soon hear from me with all the latest news, views, reviews and, er... stews?

Look, I'm tired. OK?

www.tommydonbavand.com/news

You can also email me:

mail@tommydonbavand.com

Follow me on Twitter:

www.twitter.com/tommydonbavand

And see what I'm up to on Facebook:

www.facebook.com/tommydonbavandauthor

I look forward to hearing from you!

Printed in Great Britain
by Amazon